GRACE HILL

FREESTYLE INSTANT POT COOKBOOK 2018

A Practical Approach to Watching your Weight with 100+ Easy Recipes

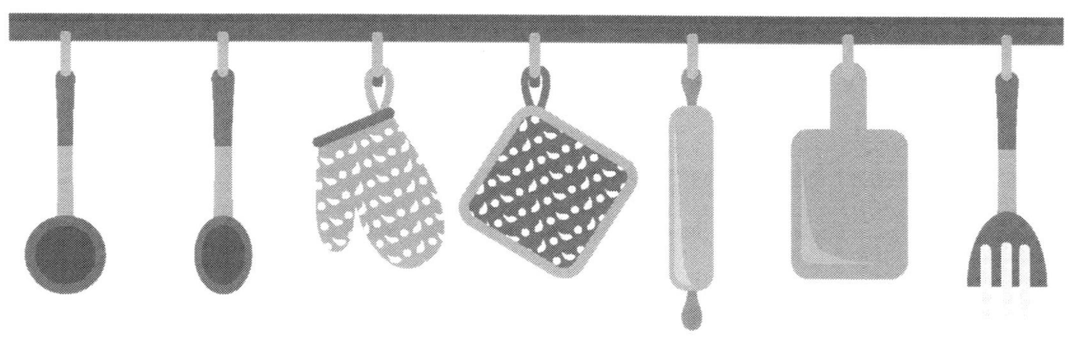

Table of Contents

Introduction

If you're one of the millions of people around the world that has ever felt self-conscious about your weight, you're not alone. Most of us (okay, *all* of us!) have experienced that dreadful feeling when your jeans won't zip quite like they used to or the generally "blah" feeling when you look in the mirror. In a world dominated by fast food, lack of exercise, and a culture that rewards missed meals or 12-hour days spent at a desk, it's no wonder that obesity is at an all-time high across the globe.

Unfortunately, losing weight is often easier said than done. While we would all love a quick fix to shed those extra pounds (and, unsurprisingly, many companies have made a small fortunate claiming as such), the fact is that real results take a bit of work. No matter what those infomercials may say, there simply aren't any pills, waist shapers, or Doctor Frankenstein-looking contraptions that can help you lose the pounds and keep them off for good.

Most diets share the same tragic, fatal flaw: focusing on what you *cannot* eat. Sure, we can all swear off sweets and salty treats for a few weeks, but it takes a very special kind of fitness junkie to completely give up these staples in our modern diets cold turkey. We've all been there: it's after midnight, your stomach is rumbling (turns out a single piece of kale and a handful of almonds actually *aren't* that satisfying), and you cave. Mid-way through your second pint of double fudge brownie ice cream, the guilt sets in as you realize that all that hard work was for nothing and you're back to square one… amidst the carnage of your latest junk food massacre.

Whether you are looking to lose weight for health reasons, an upcoming event (raise your hand if you're currently "sweating for the wedding!"), to run your first marathon, to gain a boost of confidence, or just to look fabulous in your pair of skinny jeans again, you've come to the right place. Our recipes combine the ease of Instant Pot™ cooking with the tried and true tricks of Freestyle'™ latest program: Freestyle!

Chapter 1:

A Bit About Freestyle

Close Your Eyes For a Moment...

Flashback to the mid-1990's: it's a warm summer day and hordes of people are clamoring into a small storefront shop. An old tabletop fan casually swivels in the background as, one by one, each person hops onto one of the scales that are placed in a neat little row at the far end of the room. Bubbly attendants jot down notes on their clipboards and cheerfully issue nametags to each attendee. From "Baby Weight" to "Old College Injury," the room quickly becomes a glorified melting pot of overeaters and their aptly-named pseudonyms.

Taking their seats in a small circle, it's hard to tell whether this is a scene from a dieting program or Alcoholics Anonymous. A moderator starts the show with a few chubby jokes and introduces the day's topic before each nametag-clad participant begins to share their latest dieting woes. At the end of the hour, everyone shares a cup of coffee before carrying on with their day (and calculating the points lost to that small cup of dark roast).

If this scene sounds like your own personally branded version of purgatory, we get it. After all, there's a reason that so many popular 90's sitcoms feature an episode or two about the Freestyle™ of yesteryear...

Luckily for you, our cell phones aren't the size of bricks anymore and our Freestyle™ programs have come right on into the 21st century along with those smart phones we can't live without! Gone are the days of cramped meetings, hours spent crunching points, and awkward sharing circles. Freestyle™ is now one of the most popular, modern diets in the world and it's easy to see why; one word people: results.

How Freestyle Works

Originally founded in the early 1960's, Freestyle was and still is an innovator for its time. Founded as an easier and more affordable alternative to counting calories, Freestyle™ created a program that combined accountability with an effortlessness that just wasn't available with any other diet of the time.

So, how does it all work today? While it's true that you'd barely recognize our modern day "Freestyle" compared to its older counterpart, Freestyle still relies on three main cornerstones to help you lose weight, keep those pounds off for good, and live a healthier, happier life:

- **Point System**:

  105, 231, 3. No, we're not sharing the winning combination to tonight's lottery, those numbers (however arbitrary) are the scientific calories in a single serving of banana, chicken breast, and asparagus, respectively. If, like us, math was never your best subject in grade school, then counting calories just aren't worth the hassle. The fact is that there is no rhyme or reason to the ways calories are assigned to the foods we eat, and it is nearly impossible to keep these numbers straight while still going about your business.

  Well my friends, step into the light because this is exactly why the Freestyle™ point system was created! Instead of asking you to memorize or look up some arbitrary calorie count during each and every meal, Freestyle™ does the hard work for you by assigning regularly enjoyed foods and ingredients a point value (most of which fall between 0 and 5).

  Not only does this system take the headache out of calorie counting, it also helps you subtly learn which foods are healthier than others. Put it this way, if you're trying to create a lunch of only 10 points max, you're going to want to learn which foods are worth less points (which, unsurprisingly, are your healthier options!).

- **In-Person & Virtual Meetings**:

For most people, the biggest obstacle to losing weight is themselves. After all, you didn't pick up those extra pounds by keeping yourself accountable now did you?

This is where Freestyle™ meetings come in handy. Thankfully, the days of awkward meetings are gone and meetings are now, dare we say…fun! Whether you're looking for some fresh perspectives about the Freestyle™ diet, a group of supportive friends that truly understand what you're going through during your weight loss journey, or just a bit of accountability, meetings are an excellent way to keep your diet on track.

PRO TIP: Did you know that Freestyle™ now offers an online coaching program as well? For a small additional fee, you'll be connected to your very own wellness coach that can help talk you off the edge when those cravings kick in or get to the root of your overeating!

- **Fitness & Exercise**:

Just like the foods you eat are worth points, so are the steps you take! Utilizing what the program calls FitPoints, Freestyle™ rewards you for working out! Whether you're jogging around the block, hitting the gym, or just walking to and from the office, there are points to be earned!

Chapter 2:

What Makes Freestyle Different

Ask any seasoned Freestyle™ pro what their biggest complaint was about the old program and they will tell you the same thing: point confusion. While the good ol' point system was definitely an upgrade from traditional calorie counting, it could still cause a bit of confusion. For many Freestyle™ dieters, it was hard to reconcile why a small serving of French fries had the same point value as a bowl of strawberries, or how different kinds of lettuce could be worth different points.

Well folks, as they say, the times are a changin'! The Freestyle™ Freestyle Program combines all of the benefits of the older program with one BIG change: NO Point foods! We know what you're thinking, "isn't water the only thing that has zero calories?" Technically speaking, yes you're right. But remember that we're talking points here, not calories.

Remember, the whole point of the Freestyle™ program is to encourage healthy eating which, in turn, naturally leads to weight loss. It's no coincidence that all of the NO Points foods on the Freestyle list are chock full of nutrients, each designed to help you find healthy staples in your diet for years to come! Still not convinced? Check out some of the NO Points list for yourself:

* Apples
* Apricots
* Artichoke Hearts
* Arugula
* Asparagus
* Banana
* Beans
* Broccoli
* Cabbage
* Calamari
* Carrots
* Cauliflower
* Caviar (for those moments you're particularly fancy!)
* Celery
* Chicken breast
* Coleslaw
* Corn
* Cucumber
* Dates
* Edamame
* Egg substitutes
* Egg whites
* Eggs (whole)
* Figs
* Fish
* Fruit cocktail
* Fruit cup
* Garlic
* Grapes
* Greens
* Hearts of Palm
* Jerk chicken breast
* Kiwi
* Lemon
* Lentils
* Lettuce
* Lime
* Melon
* Mushrooms
* Onions
* Passion fruit
* Peaches
* Peas
* Peppers
* Pickles
* Salad
* Sashimi
* Shellfish
* Spinach
* Tofu
* Tomatoes
* Turkey breast
* Mixed vegetables
* Watermelon
* Yogurt

That's quite a list, huh?! We challenge you to try and find one of your favorite recipes that doesn't include at least a couple of these NO Points foods (spoiler alert: it's virtually impossible)! This new approach to dieting has already helped bunches of people across the globe, so the only question left is: where can you sign up?!

Joining Freestyle

If you're completely new to the program, you'll want to start by creating an account online. Once you select the program features that are right for you, you will be able to download the Freestyle™ app to track your food points, reserve a spot in a meeting, and even track your steps!

Want more information? Visit www.weightwatchers.com today!

Chapter 3:

What Is The Instant Pot™?

A Brief History of Pressure Cookers

Think back to a time before your life was filled with a hectic schedule of staff meetings, carpools, parent-teacher conferences, and bills…a simpler time, a stress-free time. Now, as you breathe a small sigh of relief reminiscing about the good ol' days, we want you to imagine your grandmother or mother's kitchen. Remember the scrumptious smells as your grandma or mom whipped up something tasty for dinner? The aroma of a home cooked meal wafting throughout the house making your stomach growl in anticipation?

Now, how about the gadgets and gizmos your talented mom or grandma used to concoct these decadent creations? Depending on your age (don't worry, we've turned 40 a few times by now too), you may remember a strange stove-top pot used to whip up everything from baked beans to your family's secret pasta sauce. Maybe you remember the undeniable flash of her paisley-printed, lime green slow cooker or, better yet, the hours you had to wait for mom's famous chicken noodle soup.

Call them what you want, but both of these ancient kitchen tools are adaptations of the pressure cooker! Originally founded in the 1600's by Denis Papin, a French inventor and physicist, the pressure cooker has been at the top of most newlyweds' wedding registries for as long as we can remember. Why? Well, for starters, pressure cookers tend to make cooking a heck of a lot easier. Simply toss all of your ingredients into the pot, flip a switch or turn a knob, and walk away for a few hours. When you return, dinner is served!

Pressure Cooking 101

So, how exactly do pressure cookers work anyway? Great question, and the answer involves a bit of science. If chemistry and physics weren't exactly your best subjects in school, fear not! We've taken the headache out of the technicalities and break the science lingo down into plain English below:

- If you take nothing else away from this brief science lesson, listen up: pressure cookers are all about S-T-E-A-M. As the temperatures rise, so do the steam levels inside the cooker and, before long, the overall pressure increases too!
- As the pressure levels rise, the boiling point of the water also rises! Typically, the boiling point of water is 212° F but, with a pressure cooker, it increases all the way to 250° F!
- So, why do you care? Higher boiling points mean faster cooking time so you can get out of the kitchen and on with your life!
- Cooking with steam also infuses your food with added moisture for an extra juicy steak, chicken, veggie dish…you name it!

What Sets the Instant Pot™ Apart?

If you're reading this cook book, chances are pretty decent that you either already own an Instant Pot™ or have one waiting in your shopping cart as you wait to pull the trigger. If you're already a seasoned Instant Pot™ aficionado, feel free to skip ahead. But, if you're an Instant Pot™ newbie, listen up!

There's a reason the Instant Pot™ is taking the world by storm and is quickly becoming the top-selling pressure cooker available on the market today. Like all modern pressure cookers, the Instant Pot™ can cook your favorite meals in a fraction of the time. So why should you shell out a few extra bucks for an Instant Pot™ instead of that low-cost deal of the day that popped up in your inbox?

Unlike other pressure cookers out there, the Instant Pot™ can replace all of these gadgets that you may (or may not) already have collecting dust in your cabinets:

- Electric pressure cooker
- Rice cooker
- Slow cooker
- Steamer
- Warming Pot
- Browning Pan
- Most pots and pans!

Models and Gadgets and Specs, Oh My!

Another plus to cooking with an Instant Pot™ instead of some no-name pressure cooker is the assortment of models and sizes this amazing little device is available in! Right now, the Pressure Cooker comes in 5 different models and a variety of capacities to fit everyone's needs. Whether you're cooking for one or a big family of eight, there is an Instant Pot™ for you!

Need help choosing the best Instant Pot™ for you and your family? Check out the complete buyer's guide on the Instant Pot™ website

Chapter 4:

The Benefits Of Instant Pot™ Cooking

Fast Cooking Time

Remember all that mumbo-jumbo about boiling points and rising pressure levels? Well, the biggest advantage to all of that heat is a BIG benefit for you: quicker cooking time! Believe it or not, your Instant Pot™ is capable of preparing all of your favorite dishes in a mere fraction of the time. How fast are we talkin'? Imagine whipping up a chicken breast in under 10 minutes!

From rice dishes to fish, veggies to pasta, chicken to beef and everything in between, you will be absolutely shocked just how quickly your new Instant Pot™ can prepare your favorite meals! The only question left is: what will you do with all of that found time?!

Eco-Friendly

Since it prepares your food in half the time, your Instant Pot™ is also friendly to mother Earth! Not only does this nifty little device save energy, it is also made entirely out of stainless steel, which eliminates the need for those nasty non-stick chemicals that are found in most kitchen appliances. And you know what that means: less chemicals, less harm to you, less harm to the environment!

Health Conscious Eating Made Easy

Most of us can agree that healthy eating is the way to go but, sadly, that's a little bit easier said than done when you're always on the go. Sure, we would all love to spend hours upon hours in the kitchen cooking a weight loss friendly meal, but there are only so many hours in the day! This is where your Instant Pot™ comes in handy, my friends; imagine being able to enjoy all of the benefits of a healthy meal without all of the unnecessary prep, cooking, or baking time!

Chapter 5:

Freestyle + Instant Pot Cooking

Weight Loss Meets Speed

Your new Instant Pot™ and the Freestyle™ Freestyle diet are basically a match made in heaven. Think about it, Freestyle is all about making it easier to live a healthy and active lifestyle and, you guessed it, so is Instant Pot™ cooking! Both programs are dedicated to helping you live a wholesome and healthy lifestyle without unnecessary stress, so it makes sense that these two health nuts would eventually find their ways to one another sooner or later!

Endless Possibilities

Remember that seemingly endless list of NO Points foods we touched on earlier? How about all of those dishes your Instant Pot™ can prepare or the numerous other appliances it replaced? Now imagine all of the ways you can combine those NO Point foods with the dishes and features of your Instant Pot™…

Is your head spinning yet? Good! When it comes to options, the possibilities truly are limitless when you join the brand new Freestyle™ Freestyle diet with Instant Pot™ cooking. Whether you're looking for a nutritious breakfast on-the-go, a low calorie snack, or a protein-rich dinner in half the time, the sky is the limit when these two programs join forces!

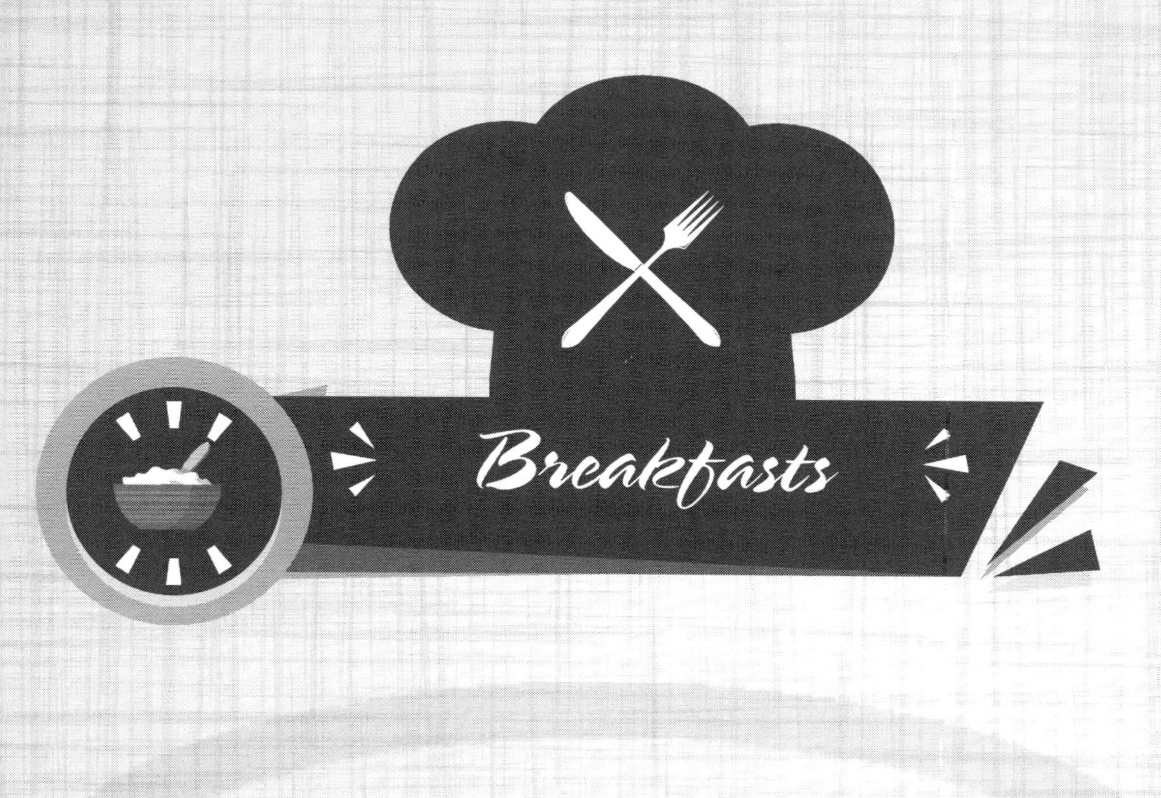
Breakfasts

Spinach Frittata

 Prep Time: 5 MIN |  Cook Time: 10 MIN |  Serves: 3

Ingredients:

For cooking:

1 tbsp olive oil

For frittata:

1 lb fresh spinach, chopped
½ cup cottage cheese, crumbled
1 small onion, chopped
4 garlic cloves, minced
2 large eggs, beaten

Seasoning:

1 tsp salt
Black pepper
Sour cream (optional)

Directions:

1. Rinse the spinach thoroughly under cold running water. Drain and chop into small pieces. Set aside.
2. In a large mixing bowl, crack the eggs and whisk until foamy and smooth. Stir in the cheese and sprinkle with some salt and pepper. Set aside.
3. Plug in the Instant Pot and grease the stainless steel insert with olive oil. Press the Sauté button and add garlic and onions. Cook for 3-4 minutes, or until the onions are translucent.
4. Add spinach and cook for 2-3 minutes, or until wilted. Pour in the eggs, spread evenly with a wooden spatula. Cook for another 3 minutes, or until the eggs are set.
5. Turn off the pot and transfer contents to a serving plate.
6. Top with some sour cream if desired and enjoy.

Freestyle Points Per Serving: 5

(Calories 172 | Total Fats 9.3g | Net Carbs: 6.7g | Protein 14.2g |Fiber: 3.9g)

Cauliflower Egg Salad

 Prep Time: 5 MIN |  Cook Time: 10 MIN | 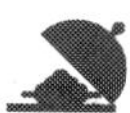 Serves: 2

Ingredients:

For cooking:

1 tbsp butter

For frittata:

1 lb cauliflower, chopped
4 large eggs
½ cup green onions, chopped
1 large tomato, wedged
½ cup cucumber, sliced

Seasoning:

1 tsp salt
½ tsp Italian seasoning
½ tsp black pepper, ground

Directions:

1. Plug in the Instant Pot and place butter in the stainless steel insert. Press Sauté button and gently stir with a wooden spatula until butter melts.
2. Add cauliflower and cook for 2 minutes. Pour 1 cup of water into pot and close the lid. Adjust the steam release handle and press the Manual button. Set the timer for 2 minutes and cook on High pressure.
3. When you hear the cookers end signal, perform a quick pressure release and open the pot. Drain the cauliflower and transfer in a large bowl. Clean the pot.
4. Set the stainless steel insert inside and pour in 2 cups of water. Gently submerge the eggs in the water and close the lid. Set the steam release handle and cook for 3 minutes on Manual mode.
5. Release the pressure naturally and open the pot.
6. Now, peel the eggs and cut into wedges. Combine with cauliflower, green onions, tomato, and cucumber. Sprinkle with salt, Italian seasoning, and pepper. Give it a good stir and serve immediately.

Freestyle Points Per Serving: 5

(Calories 142 | Total Fats 8.3g | Net Carbs: 5.9g | Protein 9.3g |Fiber: 3.9g)

Tofu Pepper Hash

 Prep Time: 5 MIN |  Cook Time: 10 MIN |  Serves: 4

Ingredients:

For cooking:

1 cup vegetable broth

For hash:

7 oz silken tofu, cut into cubes
1 large red bell pepper, chopped
1 large yellow bell pepper, chopped
1 cup button mushrooms, sliced
1 small onion, chopped
½ cup tomatoes, diced
1 tbsp olive oil

Seasoning:

1 tsp dried celery, ground
½ tsp dried thyme, ground
½ tsp garlic powder
1 tsp sea salt

Directions:

1. Plug in your Instant Pot and pour in the vegetable broth. Add tofu, bell peppers, mushrooms, and onion. Sprinkle with celery, thyme, garlic powder, and salt. Stir well and securely lock the lid.
2. Set the steam release handle and press the Manual button. Set the timer for 5 minutes and cook on High pressure.
3. When you hear the cookers end signal, perform a quick pressure release. Open the pot and stir in the tomatoes. Press the Sauté button and bring it to a boil. Simmer for 3-4 minutes, stirring occasionally.
4. Transfer contents to a serving dish and optionally, sprinkle with some fresh parsley and enjoy!

Freestyle Points Per Serving: 4

(Calories 106 | Total Fats 5.5g | Net Carbs: 7.6g | Protein 6.2g |Fiber: 1.8g)

Chicken with Asparagus

 Prep Time: 10 MIN |  Cook Time: 10 MIN | 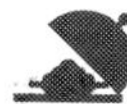 Serves: 6

Ingredients:

For cooking:

1 tbsp butter

For hash:

1 lb chicken fillets, cut into bite-sized pieces
1 lb asparagus, trimmed and chopped
1 small onion, finely chopped

For sauce:

1 tbsp mayonnaise
1 tbsp sour cream
½ tsp salt
¼ tsp dried thyme, ground
2 tsp tomato sauce
½ tsp garlic powder
¼ tsp black pepper, ground

Directions:

1. In a small bowl, combine all sauce ingredients and stir until well blended. Set aside.
2. Rinse the asparagus and trim off the woody ends. Chop into bite-sized pieces and set aside.
3. Plug in your Instant Pot and place the butter in the stainless steel insert. Gently stir until melts over Sauté mode.
4. Add chicken and sprinkle with some sea salt. Cook for 4-5 minutes, or until golden brown. Remove the chicken to a bowl, and cover.
5. Add asparagus and onions. Stir-fry for 2-3 minutes.
6. Now, return the chicken to the pot and pour in the sauce. Give it a good stir and cook for 2-3 minutes.
7. Transfer to a serving plate and serve immediately.

Freestyle Points Per Serving: 5

(Calories 196 | Total Fats 8.9g | Net Carbs: 4.2g | Protein 23.8g |Fiber: 1.9g)

Green Breakfast Puree

 Prep Time: 15 MIN |  Cook Time: 10 MIN |  Serves: 4

Ingredients:

For cooking:

1 cup chicken stock
1 tbsp olive oil

For puree:

1 lb broccoli, chopped
1 cup spinach, chopped
1 cup cauliflower, chopped
1 medium-sized red onion, finely chopped
2 garlic cloves, minced

Seasoning:

1 tsp salt
½ tsp black pepper, ground
¼ tsp red pepper flakes
¼ tsp dried marjoram, ground

Directions:

1. Plug in the Instant Pot and grease the stainless steel insert with olive oil. Add onions and garlic. Stir-fry for 3-4 minutes, or until translucent.
2. Add broccoli, spinach, and cauliflower. Sprinkle with some salt and pepper. Pour in the chicken stock and stir well.
3. Securely lock the lid and adjust the steam release handle. Press the Manual button and set the steam release handle. Set the timer for 5 minutes and cook on High pressure.
4. When done, perform a quick pressure release and open the pot. Let it chill for a while.
5. Transfer all to a food processor and blend until smooth. Transfer to a serving dish and sprinkle with some red pepper flakes and dried marjoram.
6. Optionally, serve with some whole wheat bread.

Freestyle Points Per Serving: 3

(Calories 93 | Total Fats 4.1g | Net Carbs: 8.1g | Protein 4.5g |Fiber: 4.5g)

Fried Vegetables

 Prep Time: 15 MIN |  Cook Time: 10 MIN |  Serves: 3

Ingredients:

For cooking:
1 tbsp olive oil

For puree :
2 red bell peppers, sliced
1 yellow bell pepper, sliced
1 small onion, finely chopped
1 cup cauliflower, cut into florets
2 baby carrots, sliced
1 cup button mushrooms, sliced
¼ cup celery root, finely chopped
1 garlic clove, crushed

Seasoning:
1 tsp salt
½ tsp black pepper
½ tsp dried thyme
¼ tsp dried rosemary

Directions:

1. Plug in the Instant Pot and press the Sauté button. Grease the inner pot with olive oil and add cauliflower, carrots, and garlic. Sprinkle with salt and give it a good stir. Cook for 3-4 minutes, stirring occasionally.
2. Now add celery root, onions, and bell peppers. Continue to cook for 5-6 minutes, or until vegetables have softened.
3. Finally, add mushrooms and season with some more salt, pepper, thyme, and rosemary. Pour in about ¼ cup of water and stir all well.
4. Cook until all the liquid has evaporated.
5. Remove from the heat and serve immediately.

Freestyle Points Per Serving: 4

(Calories 110 | Total Fats 5.2g | Net Carbs: 12.2g | Protein 3.2g |Fiber: 3.6g)

Scrambled Eggs with Salmon

 Prep Time: 15 MIN |  Cook Time: 10 MIN |  Serves: 4

Ingredients:

For cooking:

1 tbsp olive oil
1 cup fish stock

For scrambled eggs:

7oz salmon fillet
4 eggs
2 spring onions, finely chopped
1 leek, chopped
2 garlic cloves, crushed

Seasoning:

1 tsp salt
1 tbsp fresh dill
½ tsp red pepper flakes

Directions:

1. Plug in the Instant Pot and pour in the fish stock in the inner pot. Add salmon and sprinkle with some salt.
2. Seal the lid and set the steam release handle to the Sealing position. Press the Manual button and set the timer for 5 minutes on High pressure.
3. When done, perform a quick pressure release and open the lid. Remove the salmon and transfer to a cutting board. Using a sharp knife, chop the fillet into bite-sized pieces and set aside.
4. Now, press the Sauté button. Heat up the oil and add leeks and garlic. Cook for 4-5 minutes, stirring constantly.
5. Add spring onions and chopped salmon. Season with more salt and pepper. Give it a good stir and continue to cook for another 5 minutes.
6. Finally, add eggs and stir all well. Cook for 1-2 minutes.
7. Remove from the pot and sprinkle with fresh dill. Serve immediately.

Freestyle Points Per Serving: 5

(Calories 187 | Total Fats 11.5g | Net Carbs: 3.9g | Protein 17.1g |Fiber: 0.6g)

Creamy Broccoli

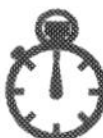 Prep Time: 10 MIN | 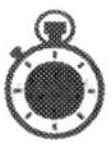 Cook Time: 10 MIN | 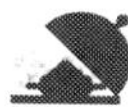 Serves: 4

Ingredients:

For cooking:

2 cups vegetable stock

For broccoli :

1 lb broccoli, chopped
1 cup Brussels sprouts, halved
1 medium-sized red onion, sliced
2 garlic cloves, minced
½ tsp salt

For the sauce:

1 tbsp soy sauce
2 tbsp heavy cream
1 tbsp olive oil
1 tsp fresh lime juice
½ tsp black pepper, ground
½ tsp salt
¼ tsp ginger, freshly ground

Directions:

1. Combine broccoli and Brussels sprouts in the stainless steel insert of your Instant Pot. Pour in the stock and sprinkle with some salt. Securely lock the lid and adjust the steam release handle by moving the valve to the Sealing position. Press the Manual button and set the timer for 5 minutes. Cook on High pressure.
2. When done, perform a quick pressure release and open the pot. Remove the vegetables using a large slotted spoon.
3. In a food processor, combine onions, garlic, and all sauce ingredients. Blend until smooth and creamy.
4. Press the Sauté button and add all sauce ingredients. Cook for 5 minutes, or until sauce thickens. Stir occasionally.
5. Pour the sauce over cooked vegetables and serve immediately.

Freestyle Points Per Serving: 4

(Calories 123 | Total Fats 6.8g | Net Carbs: 9g | Protein 5g |Fiber: 4.8g)

Kohlrabi Chicken

 Prep Time: 15 MIN |  Cook Time: 15 MIN | 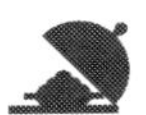 Serves: 6

Ingredients:

For cooking:

2 tsp olive oil

For kohlrabi chicken :

1 lb chicken breasts, skinless and boneless
2 cups kohlrabi, chopped into bite-sized pieces
1 medium-sized red bell pepper, chopped
1 small onion, chopped
2 garlic cloves, finely chopped
1 small chili pepper, chopped

Seasoning:

1 tsp sea salt
½ tsp dried thyme, ground
½ tsp cayenne pepper, ground
¼ tsp black pepper, ground

Directions:

1. Rinse the meat thoroughly under running water and pat dry with a kitchen paper. Generously rub with salt, cayenne pepper, and black pepper. Set aside.
2. Wash the kohlrabi and trim off the green ends. Cut into bite-sized pieces and set aside.
3. Plug in the Instant Pot and grease the stainless steel with olive oil. Press the Sauté button and add chicken breasts. Cook for 3 minutes on each side. Remove the breasts to a plate and set aside.
4. Add onions, garlic, and red chili pepper. Cook for 2-3 minutes and add kohlrabi chops. Stir well and pour 1 cup of water. Securely lock the lid and adjust the steam release handle. Press the Manual button and cook for 5 minutes on High pressure.
5. When you hear the cookers end signal, perform a quick pressure release and open the pot.
6. Place the chicken on a serving plate and top with cooked kohlrabi.

Freestyle Points Per Serving: 4

(Calories 182 | Total Fats 7.3g | Net Carbs: 3.6g | Protein 23g |Fiber: 2.2g)

Trout Brussels Sprout Hash

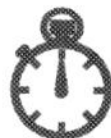 Prep Time: 15 MIN |  Cook Time: 15 MIN |  Serves: 6

Ingredients:

For cooking:

2 tsp butter

For hash:

1 lb trout fillets, cut into bite-sized pieces
1 lb Brussels sprouts, chopped
2 medium-sized carrots, chopped
1 large turnip, chopped
3 large eggs

Seasoning:

1 tsp sea salt
1 tsp dried parsley, ground
¼ tsp dried dill, ground
½ tsp Italian seasoning

Directions:

1. Plug in the Instant Pot and place butter in the stainless steel insert. Press the Saute button and gently stir, until butter melts.
2. Add chopped trout and sprinkle with some salt. Cook for 3-4 minutes, stirring occasionally.
3. Now, add Brussels sprouts, carrots, and turnips. Add water enough to cover and sprinkle with dried parsley, dill, and Italian seasoning. Stir well and close the lid. Set the steam release handle and press the Manual button. Set the timer for 7 minutes and cook on High pressure.
4. When you hear the cookers end signal, perform a quick pressure release and open the pot. Drain the ingredients and return to the pot.
5. Press the Sauté button and poach the eggs on top. Cook for 2 more minutes, or until the eggs are set.
6. Transfer all to a serving plate and enjoy!

Freestyle Points Per Serving: 6

(Calories 240 | Total Fats 10.5g | Net Carbs: 8.9g | Protein 26.3g |Fiber: 3.9g)

Mushroom Pepper Quiche

 Prep Time: 15 MIN |  Cook Time: 17 MIN |  Serves: 6

Ingredients:

For cooking:

2 tsp olive oil

For quiche:

2 cups button mushrooms, sliced
1 large red bell pepper, chopped
1 large green bell pepper, diced
2 cups fresh spinach, chopped
6 eggs, beaten
¼ cup milk, fat-free

Seasoning:

1 tsp sea salt
½ tsp black pepper, ground
1 tsp dried thyme, ground

Directions:

1. Line a fitting spring-form pan with some parchment paper and grease the walls with some cooking spray. Set aside.

1. Plug in the Instant Pot and grease the stainless steel insert with olive oil. Add mushrooms and bell peppers. Cook for 3-4 minutes, stirring occasionally.
2. Add spinach and continue to cook for 3 more minutes or until spinach is wilted. Transfer all to a prepared spring-form pan.
3. In a large mixing bowl, combine eggs, and remaining spices. Lightly whisk and pour over the vegetables.
4. Add 1 cup of water to the pot and set the trivet on the bottom. Place the pan on top and securely lock the lid.
5. Set the steam release handle by moving the valve to the Sealing position. Press the Manual button and cook for 10 minutes on High pressure.
6. When done, perform a quick pressure release and open the pot. Carefully transfer the pan to a wire rack and let it chill for a while.
7. Optionally, sprinkle with some chives before serving. Enjoy!

Freestyle Points Per Serving: 3

(Calories 101 | Total Fats 6.4g | Net Carbs: 4g | Protein 7.3g |Fiber: 1g)

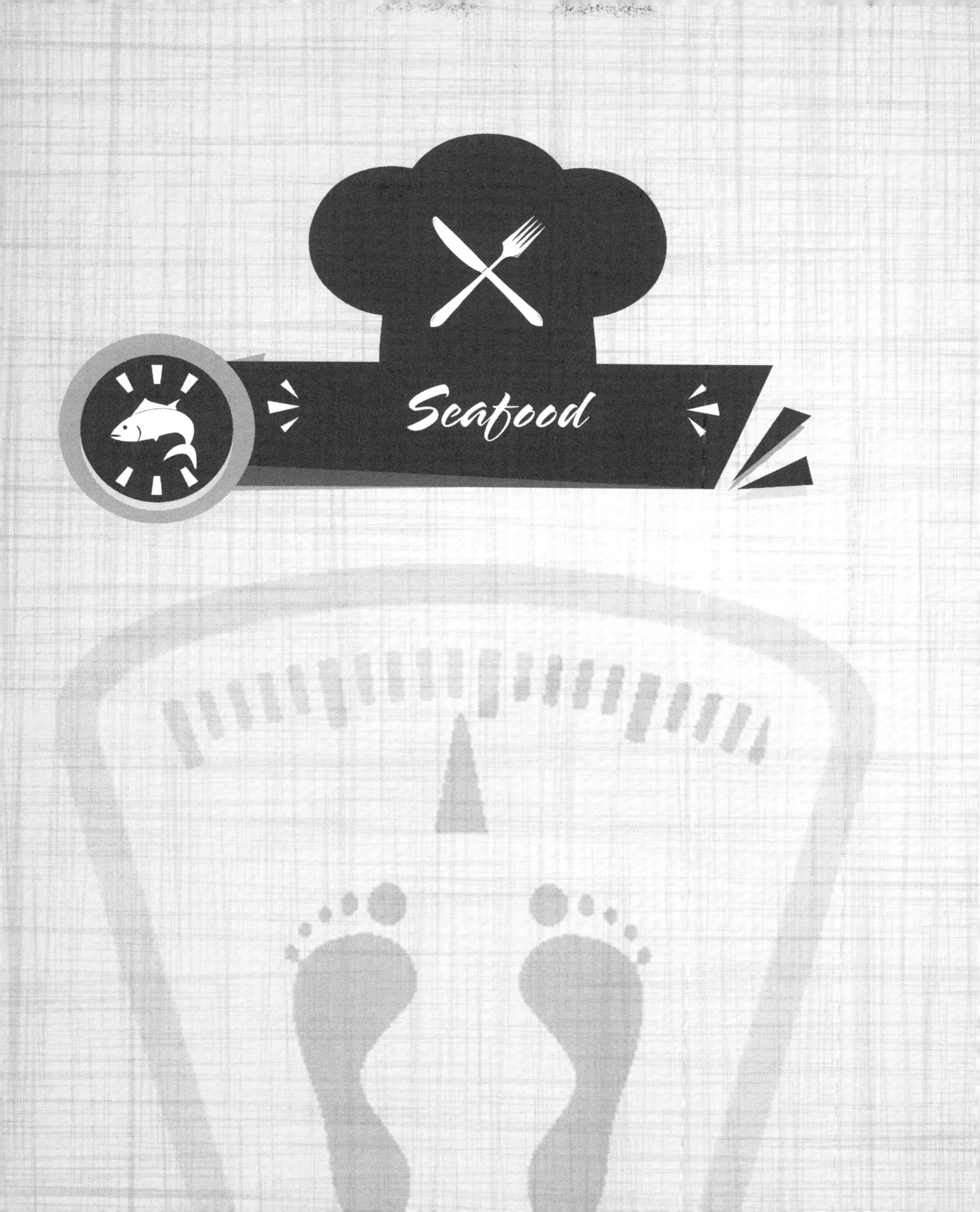
Seafood

Shrimp Scampi with Cucumber Dill Sauce

 Prep Time: 5 MIN |  Cook Time: 7 MIN | 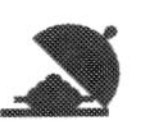 Serves: 2

Ingredients:

For cooking:

Nonstick spray

For shrimp scampi:

4 oz shrimps, cleaned and deveined
½ cup broccoli, chopped
1 small carrot, sliced
1 small onion, finely chopped
1 garlic clove, finely chopped
½ tsp sea salt
¼ tsp cayenne pepper, ground

For cucumber dill sauce:

½ cup cucumber, sliced
1 tsp mayonnaise, fat-free
1 tsp fresh dill, finely chopped
½ tsp garlic powder
¼ tsp dried thyme, ground
½ tsp salt
½ tsp black pepper, ground

Directions:

1. In a food processor or a blender, combine cucumber, mayonnaise, dill, garlic powder, dried thyme, salt, and pepper. Pulse until smooth and creamy. Set aside.
2. Plug in your Instant Pot and press the Sauté button. Spray with some non-stick cooking spray and add onions and garlic. Stir-fry for 3-4 minutes, or until the onions are translucent. Add shrimps and sprinkle with sea salt and cayenne pepper. Cook for 1 minute, turning once.
3. Add broccoli and carrot. Securely lock the lid and adjust the steam release handle. Press the Manual button and cook for 2 minutes on High pressure.
4. When done, perform a quick pressure release and open the pot. Drain the ingredients and transfer to a large colander.
5. Drizzle with cucumber dill sauce and serve immediately. Enjoy!

Freestyle Points Per Serving: 6

(Calories 242 | Total Fats 4g | Net Carbs: 17.9g | Protein 29.5g |Fiber: 5g)

Sweet Apple Trout

 Prep Time: 5 MIN |  Cook Time: 4 MIN | 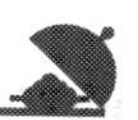 Serves: 4

Ingredients:

For cooking:

1 tsp sesame oil

For shrimp scampi:

7 oz trout fillets, cut into bite-sized pieces
1 medium-sized Granny Smiths apple, cut into bite-sized pieces
1 tsp soy sauce
1 tsp rice vinegar
1 tsp lemon juice, freshly squeezed

Seasoning:

½ tsp sea salt
1 tbsp fresh parsley, finely chopped
½ tsp black pepper, ground
¼ tsp dried rosemary, ground

Directions:

1. In a large bowl, combine soy sauce, rice vinegar, lemon juice, sea salt, parsley, black pepper, and rosemary. Mix until combined and brush the fish with this mixture.
2. Plug in the Instant Pot and grease the stainless steel insert with sesame oil. Press the Sauté button and add fish and apple. Cook for 2 minutes, stirring occasionally.
3. Add enough water to cover and securely lock the lid. Adjust the steam release handle and press the Manual button. Set the timer for 2 minutes and cook on High pressure.
4. When you hear the cookers end signal, perform a quick pressure release by turning the valve to the Venting position. Open the pot and transfer to a serving plate. Enjoy!

Freestyle Points Per Serving: 3

(Calories 126 | Total Fats 5.3g | Net Carbs: 4.3g | Protein 13.3g |Fiber: 1.3g)

Spicy Salmon with Apricot Salsa

 Prep Time: 10 MIN |  Cook Time: 8 MIN | 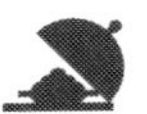 Serves: 4

Ingredients:

For cooking:

1 tsp avocado oil

For salmon:

1 lb salmon fillets, cut into 4 equal pieces
1 small onion, finely chopped
1 garlic clove, minced
1 tsp sea salt
¼ tsp red pepper chili flakes
¼ tsp cayenne pepper, ground

For apricot salsa:

2 large apricots, pitted
½ tsp sea salt
1 tbsp fresh parsley, finely chopped
½ tsp black pepper, ground
¼ tsp dried rosemary, ground

Directions:

1. First, prepare the apricot salsa: simply combine all salsa ingredients in a food processor and blend until smooth. Set aside.
2. Plug in the Instant Pot and grease the stainless steel insert with some avocado oil. Add onions, garlic, red chili pepper flakes, and cayenne pepper. Stir-fry for 2 minutes and add salmon fillets. Cook for 2 minutes on each side and remove from the pot.
3. Pour the salsa into the pot and add 2-3 tbsp of water. Close the lid and adjust the steam release handle by moving the valve to the Sealing position. Cook for 2 minutes over Manual mode on High pressure.
4. When done, perform a quick pressure release and open the pot.
5. Drizzle the salsa over salmon fillets and serve immediately. Enjoy!

Freestyle Points Per Serving: 5

(Calories 169 | Total Fats 7.3g | Net Carbs: 3.3g | Protein 22.6g |Fiber: 0.9g)

Salmon Risotto

 Prep Time: 5 MIN |  Cook Time: 10 MIN |  Serves: 3

Ingredients:

For cooking:

2 tsp olive oil

For risotto:

1 cup cauliflower florets, finely chopped
7 oz salmon fillets
1 large tomato, roughly chopped
1 red bell pepper, sliced
¼ cup green peas
2 medium-sized celery stalk, chopped

Seasoning:

2 tsp Cajun seasoning
½ tsp white pepper, ground

Directions:

1. Plug in the Instant Pot and add olive oil to the stainless steel insert. Heat on Sauté mode and add salmon, tomato, red bell pepper, green peas, and celery. Stir-fry for 3-4 minutes and then add 1 cup of water.
2. Bring it to a boil and add cauliflower. Cook for 5 more minutes, stirring occasionally.
3. Sprinkle with Cajun seasoning and white pepper. Optionally, add some salt and chili pepper for spicier taste.
4. Turn off the pot and transfer to a serving plate.
5. Optionally, sprinkle with some fresh chives or finely chopped spring onions. Enjoy!

Freestyle Points Per Serving: 4

(Calories 160 | Total Fats 7.5g | Net Carbs: 6.6g | Protein 15.3g |Fiber: 3.1g)

Sea Bream Patties

 Prep Time: 15 MIN | 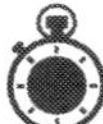 Cook Time: 8 MIN |  Serves: 4

Ingredients:

For cooking:

Nonstick cooking spray

For patties:

1 lb sea bream fillets, finely chopped
¼ cup Greek yogurt, fat-free
1 small onion, finely chopped
3 tbsp all-purpose flour
2 tbsp fresh parsley, finely chopped
1 tsp baking soda

Seasoning:

Salt
Black pepper

Directions:

1. In a large mixing bowl, combine fish, Greek yogurt, onion, flour, parsley, and baking soda. Season with some salt and pepper. Optionally, add some more herbs such as dried thyme, rosemary, or marjoram. Mix well and form 6 equal balls. Gently press each with the palms of your hands to flatten. Set aside.
2. Plug in the Instant Pot and grease the stainless steel insert with some cooking spray. Press the Sauté button and add patties.
3. Cook for 3-4 minutes on each side.
4. Serve the sea bream patties with some fat-free yogurt or fresh salad. Enjoy!

Freestyle Points Per Serving: 3

(Calories 183 | Total Fats 5.8g | Net Carbs: 5.9g | Protein 24.3g |Fiber: 0.6g)

Thai Green Curry

 Prep Time: 10 MIN |  Cook Time: 1 HOUR 5 MIN | 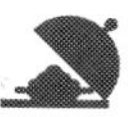 Serves: 5

Ingredients:

For cooking:

1 tsp coconut oil

For curry:

7 oz shrimps, cleaned and deveined

2 tbsp green curry paste

¾ cup coconut milk, reduced fat

½ cup bamboo shoot, chopped

2 green chilies, chopped

4 tsp fish sauce

4 tbsp Thai basil leaves

Seasoning:

½ tsp red pepper flakes

½ tsp salt

Directions:

1. Plug in the Instant Pot and add coconut oil to the stainless steel insert. Press the Sauté button and gently stir with a wooden spatula, until oil melts.
2. Add shrimps, bamboo shoots, and green chilies. Cook for 2 minutes, stirring constantly.
3. Now, add 2 tbsp coconut milk, fish sauce, and basil. Stir in the green curry paste and cook for 1 minute more.
4. Add the remaining milk and pour in ¾ cup of water. Sprinkle with salt and pepper.
5. Securely lock the lid and adjust the steam release handle. Set the Slow Cooker mode and set the timer for 1 hour.
6. When you hear the cookers end signal, release the pressure naturally.
7. Open the pot and transfer to a serving bowl. Enjoy with a side serving of rice if desired!

Freestyle Points Per Serving: 7

(Calories 163 | Total Fats 11.5g | Net Carbs: 4.4g | Protein 10.5g |Fiber: 1.2g)

Crab Parsley Patties

 Prep Time: 15 MIN |  Cook Time: 13 MIN | 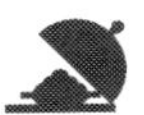 Serves: 6

Ingredients:

For cooking:

Nonstick cooking spray

For patties:

1 lb crab meat

½ cup fresh parsley, finely chopped

1 small red onion, finely chopped

3 large eggs, lightly beaten

2 tsp dry sherry

½ cup panko breadcrumbs

1 tsp butter

Seasoning:

1 tsp salt

¼ tsp black pepper, ground

¼ tsp garlic powder

Directions:

1. Plug in the Instant Pot and press the Sauté button. Add butter and gently stir with a wooden spatula until melts.
2. Add onions and stir-fry for 4-5 minutes, or until lightly caramelized. Remove to a large bowl and turn off the pot.
3. Add crab meat, parsley, eggs, sherry, salt, pepper, and garlic powder to the bowl with onions. Mix well with your hands and form the patties, about 3-inch in diameter. Roll in breadcrumbs and transfer to baking sheet. Refrigerate for 20 minutes.
4. Spray the inner pot with some cooking spray and press the Sauté button. Cook patties 3-4 minutes on each side, or until nicely browned. Enjoy!

Freestyle Points Per Serving: 5

(Calories 155 | Total Fats 4.1g | Net Carbs: 13.5g | Protein 9.4g |Fiber: 0.8g)

Mackerel in Tartar Sauce

 Prep Time: 10 MIN | 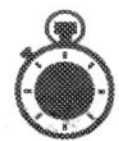 Cook Time: 6 MIN |  Serves: 8

Ingredients:

For cooking:

Nonstick cooking spray

For mackerel:

2 lbs mackerel fillets, thinly sliced
2 tbsp fresh lemon juice
3 tsp olive oil
1 tsp sea salt
½ tsp dried thyme, ground

For tartar sauce:

2 tbsp pickles, finely chopped
1 tbsp capers, finely chopped
1 tbsp mayonnaise, fat-free
¼ tsp sugar
1 tsp onion powder
¼ tsp garlic powder
½ tsp dried dill, ground

Directions:

1. In a medium-sized mixing bowl, combine mayonnaise, sugar, onion, powder, garlic powder, and dried dill. Mix until combined and then add pickles and capers. Mix again and cover with a lid. Refrigerate til later.
2. Rinse the fish fillets under cold running water. Pat dry with a kitchen paper and place in a large bowl. Drizzle with lemon juice and olive oil. Sprinkle with salt and dried thyme. Gently rub with your hands to coat all. Refrigerate for 20 minutes before cooking.
3. Grease the stainless steel insert of your Instant Pot with some cooking spray. Press the Sauté button and add fillets. Cook for 2-3 minutes on each side.
4. Optionally, add 1 cup of water and close the lid. Adjust the steam release handle and press the Manual button. Set the timer for 3 minutes and cook on High pressure.
5. When done, perform a quick pressure release and open the pot.
6. Transfer the fish to a serving plate and drizzle with tartar sauce. Enjoy!

Freestyle Points Per Serving: 8

(Calories 316 | Total Fats 22g | Net Carbs: 0.6g | Protein 27.2g |Fiber: 0.1g)

Worcestershire Halibut

 Prep Time: 5 MIN |  Cook Time: 4 MIN | 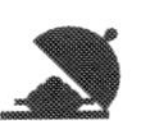 Serves: 4

Ingredients:

For cooking:

Nonstick cooking spray

For Worcestershire halibut:

8 oz halibut fillets
2 tsp Worcestershire sauce
4 tsp Dijon mustard
1 tsp fresh lime juice
½ cup fish stock

Seasoning:

½ tsp salt
½ tsp black pepper, ground
¼ tsp dried rosemary, ground

Directions:

1. Rinse the halibut fillets under running water and pat dry with a kitchen paper. Rub the salt, pepper, and rosemary with your hands. Set aside.
2. In a mixing bowl, combine Worcestershire sauce, Dijon mustard, and lime juice. Mix until well combined
3. Plug in the Instant Pot and spray the stainless steel insert with some nonstick cooking spray. When heated, add the fish and brush with previously prepared mixture. Press the Sauté button and cook for 1 minute on each side.
4. Pour in the fish stock and securely lock the lid. Adjust the steam release handle and press the Manual button. Set the timer for 2 minutes. Cook on High pressure.
5. When you hear the cookers end signal, perform a quick pressure release and open the pot. Transfer the fish to a serving plate and garnish with some lime slices and finely chopped parsley.

Freestyle Points Per Serving: 3

(Calories 251 | Total Fats 4.4g | Net Carbs: 0.6g | Protein 46.9g |Fiber: 0.2g)

Steamed Trout with Tomatoes

 Prep Time: 10 MIN | 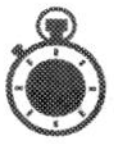 Cook Time: 34 MIN |  Serves: 4

Ingredients:

For cooking:

Nonstick cooking spray

For trout:

1 lb trout fillets
2 tsp olive oil
1 tsp fresh rosemary, finely chopped
¼ tsp garlic powder
½ tsp smoked salt

For tomatoes:

1 large tomato, sliced
1 small onion, thinly sliced
½ tsp dried oregano, ground
¼ tsp dried marjoram, ground

Directions:

1. Plug in the Instant Pot and pour 1 cup of water in the stainless steel insert.
2. Place the fish in the steam basket and sprinkle with olive oil, rosemary, garlic, and salt.
3. Position a trivet on the bottom of your Instant Pot and place the steam basket on top. Securely lock the lid and adjust the steam release handle. Press the Steam button and set the timer for 30 minutes.
4. When you hear the cookers end signal, release the pressure naturally.
5. Open the pot and remove the basket. Clean the pot and pat dry with a kitchen paper.
6. Now, grease the stainless steel insert with some cooking spray. Add onions and tomatoes. Sprinkle with oregano and marjoram. Stir-fry for 2-3 minutes, or until onions lightly translucent. Add fish and cook for 1 minute on each side.
7. Transfer to a serving plate and enjoy!

Freestyle Points Per Serving: 5

(Calories 253 | Total Fats 12.1g | Net Carbs: 2.7g | Protein 30.9g |Fiber: 1.2g)

Garlic Shrimps with Broccoli

 Prep Time: 5 MIN |  Cook Time: 7 MIN | 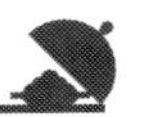 Serves: 4

Ingredients:

For cooking:

1 cup fish stock
1 tsp coconut oil

For garlic shrimps:

1 lb shrimps, peeled and deveined
4 garlic cloves, finely chopped
1 tsp fresh ginger, grated
1 tsp cornstarch
2 tbsp soy sauce, low-sodium
1 medium-sized red onion, finely chopped
½ tsp salt

For broccoli:

1 cup broccoli, chopped into florets
½ tsp Italian seasoning
¼ tsp red pepper flakes

Directions:

1. Plug in the Instant Pot and pour the fish stock in the stainless steel insert. Add broccoli and sprinkle with Italian seasoning and red pepper flakes. Securely lock the lid and set the steam release handle. Cook for 2 minutes using the Manual mode on High pressure.
2. When done, perform a quick pressure release and open the pot. Drain the broccoli and transfer to a bowl. Cover with a lid and set aside. Reserve the fish stock.
3. Now, add shrimps and close the lid again. Set the steam release handle and press the Manual button. Set the timer for 1 minute and cook on High pressure.
4. When done, open the pot and press the Sauté button. Add garlic, onions, and ginger. Stir-fry for 1 minute and then stir in the cornstarch and soy sauce. Continue to cook for another 2-3 minutes or until the sauce thickens. Sprinkle with some salt and give it a good stir. Turn off the pot.
5. Serve creamy shrimps with broccoli and enjoy!

Freestyle Points Per Serving: 4

(Calories 186 | Total Fats 3.7g | Net Carbs: 7g | Protein 28.8g |Fiber: 1.4g)

Poultry

Salsa Verde Chicken

 Prep Time: 15 MIN |  Cook Time: 18 MIN |  Serves: 0

Ingredients:

For cooking:

Nonstick spray

For chicken:

2 lbs chicken fillets, thinly sliced
½ cup green peas, frozen
1 medium-sized onion, chopped
½ tsp salt
¼ tsp black pepper, ground
¼ tsp dried thyme, ground

For salsa verde sauce:

4 tsp extra virgin olive oil
2 tsp red wine vinegar
½ tsp garlic powder
2 tbsp fresh basil, finely chopped
2 tbsp fresh parsley, final chopped
1 tbsp fresh mint, finely chopped
2 tsp capers, reduced sodium
2 anchovies, reduced sodium
1 tsp Dijon mustard
½ tsp sea salt
½ tsp black pepper, ground

Directions:

1. In a small mixing bowl, combine all salsa verde ingredients. Mix until well combined and set aside.
2. Rinse the fillets under running water. Pat dry with a kitchen paper and sprinkle with some salt, pepper and thyme. Set aside.
   Plug in the Instant Pot and grease the stainless steel insert with some cooking spray. Press the Sauté button and heat up the pot. Add onions and cook for 3-4 minutes, or until the onions are translucent. Add chicken fillets and cook for 3-4 minutes on each side. Remove from the pot.
3. Add beans and pour 1 cup of water. Securely lock the lid and adjust the steam release handle. Press the Manual button and set the timer for 8 minutes on High pressure.
4. When done, perform a quick pressure release and open the pot.
5. Serve chicken with peas and drizzle with some salsa verde sauce.
6. Enjoy!

Freestyle Points Per Serving: 5

(Calories 261 | Total Fats 11.3g | Net Carbs: 2.1g | Protein 35.1g |Fiber: 0.9g)

Chicken Mini Quiche

 Prep Time: 10 MIN |  Cook Time: 20 MIN | 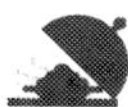 Serves: 3

Ingredients:

For cooking:
Nonstick spray

For quiche:
3.5 oz chicken breast, skinless, boneless, and cut into bite-sized pieces
5 large eggs
½ cup heavy cream
1 cup cottage cheese
3 tbsp fresh parsley, finely chopped

Seasoning:
1 tsp fresh thyme, ground
½ tsp cayenne pepper, ground
½ tsp salt

Directions:

1. In a large mixing bowl, whisk the eggs, heavy cream, and cottage cheese. Add finely chopped parsley, thyme, cayenne pepper, and salt. Finally, add chicken and stir until all well combined.
2. Sprinkle 2 small mini tart pans with some cooking spray. Pour in the quiche mixture and set aside.
3. Plug in the Instant Pot and pour 1 cup of water into the stainless steel insert. Position a trivet on the bottom and set the tarts on top. Securely lock the lid and adjust the steam release handle by moving the valve to the Sealing position.
4. Press the Manual button and set the timer for 20 minutes on High pressure.
5. When done, perform a quick pressure release. Move the top valve to the Venting position. Open the pot and carefully transfer the pans to a wire rack.
6. Let it cool for a while. Enjoy!

Freestyle Points Per Serving: 8

(Calories 295 | Total Fats 18g | Net Carbs: 4.1g | Protein 28.4g |Fiber: 0.1g)

Chicken Thighs with Onions

 Prep Time: 10 MIN |  Cook Time: 30 MIN | 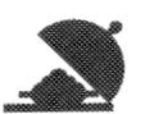 Serves: 4

Ingredients:

For cooking:

2 tsp olive oil

For chicken wings:

4 chicken thighs, skinless and boneless
1 medium-sized purple onion, sliced
1 garlic clove, crushed
2 tbsp fresh lemon juice

Seasoning:

1 tsp red chili powder
1 tsp garlic powder
Salt
Black pepper

Directions:

1. Line a fitting spring-form pan with some parchment paper and set aside.
2. In a small mixing bowl, combine olive oil, lemon juice, chili powder, garlic powder, salt, and pepper. Stir until well blended.
3. Brush the chicken thighs with the previously prepared mixture and place in the spring-form pan along with sliced onion and garlic.
4. Plug in the Instant Pot and pour 1 cup of water in the stainless steel insert. Set the trivet on the bottom and place the pan on top.
5. Securely lock the lid and adjust the steam release handle. Press the Manual button and set the timer for 30 minutes. Cook on High pressure.
6. When done, perform a quick pressure release and open the pot. Using oven mitts, transfer the pan to a wire rack and let chicken cool for a while.
7. Optionally, sprinkle with some fresh parsley before serving. Enjoy!

Freestyle Points Per Serving: 6

(Calories 311 | Total Fats 13.2g | Net Carbs: 2.4g | Protein 42.7g |Fiber: 0.6g)

Turkey Breasts with Asparagus

 Prep Time: 20 MIN |  Cook Time: 15 MIN |  Serves: 4

Ingredients:

For cooking:

Nonstick cooking spray

For turkey breasts:

1 lb turkey breasts, skinless and boneless
1 tbsp dry red wine
2 tsp fresh lime juice
4 tbsp chicken broth, reduced sodium
1 tbsp olive oil
½ tsp dried thyme, ground
¼ tsp dried rosemary, ground
½ tsp sea salt

For asparagus:

1 cup asparagus, trimmed and cut into bite-sized pieces
1 tsp butter
½ tsp Italian seasoning
¼ tsp black pepper, ground

Directions:

1. In a large bowl, combine dry red wine, lime juice, chicken broth, olive oil, thyme, rosemary, and salt. Mix until combined and then add chicken fillets. Coat well with marinade and refrigerate for at least 30 minutes.
2. Plug in the Instant Pot and spray the stainless steel insert with some nonstick cooking spray. Press the Sauté button and add drained fillets. Reserve the marinade for later.
3. Cook for 3-4 minutes on each side and remove from the pot.
4. Now, melt the butter and add asparagus. Sprinkle with Italian seasoning and pepper. Cook for 2 minutes and then pour 1 cup of water. Securely lock the lid and adjust the steam release handle. Press the Manual button and cook for 2 minutes on High pressure.
5. When done, perform a quick pressure release and open the pot. Pour in the reserved marinade and press Sauté button. Stir in 1 tbsp all-purpose flour and cook for 4-5 minutes, or until the sauce thickens to the desired consistency.
6. Serve turkey breasts with creamy asparagus and enjoy!

Freestyle Points Per Serving: 4

(Calories 156 | Total Fats 5.5g | Net Carbs: 5.4g | Protein 19.7g |Fiber: 4.2g)

Chicken Wok in Ginger Gravy

 Prep Time: 15 MIN |  Cook Time: 14 MIN |  Serves: 6

Ingredients:

For cooking:

Nonstick cooking spray

For wok:

1 lb chicken breasts, skinless and boneless
1 red bell pepper, cut into strips
½ cup broccoli, chopped
½ cup cauliflower, chopped

For ginger gravy:

1 tbsp fresh ginger, grated
1 tbsp dry sherry
2 tsp soy sauce, reduced sodium
1 tsp coconut sugar
2 tbsp fresh lemon juice
2 tsp coconut oil, melted
¼ cup chicken stock, reduced sodium

Directions:

1. In a medium-sized mixing bowl, combine all ginger gravy ingredients. Mix until well combined and set aside.

1. Plug in the Instant Pot and grease the stainless steel insert with nonstick cooking spray. Add chicken breasts and optionally, sprinkle with some salt. Cook for 3 minutes on each side, or until lightly browned. Transfer to a cutting board and cut into bite-sized pieces. Place in a bowl and cover with a lid. Set aside.
2. Now, add bell pepper, broccoli and cauliflower to the pot. Pour enough water to cover and securely lock the lid. Adjust the steam release handle and press the Manual button. Set the timer for 3 minutes and cook on High pressure.
3. When done, perform a quick pressure release. Drain the vegetables and remove the liquid. Return the vegetables to the pot and add chicken.
4. Press the Sauté button and pour in the gravy. Bring it to a boil and cook for 4-5 minutes, stirring occasionally.
5. Transfer to serving bowls and optionally, sprinkle with some finely chopped green onions.

Freestyle Points Per Serving: 4

(Calories 176 | Total Fats 7.3g | Net Carbs: 2.6g | Protein 22.7g |Fiber: 0.8g)

Chicken Broccoli Linguine

 Prep Time: 20 MIN | 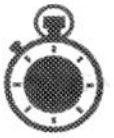 Cook Time: 13 MIN |  Serves: 5

Ingredients:

For cooking:

2 tsp olive oil

For chicken broccoli:

1 lb chicken fillets, cut into bite-sized pieces
1 cup broccoli, chopped into florets
1 tsp soy sauce, reduced sodium
2 tbsp chicken broth, reduced sodium
½ tsp garlic powder
½ tsp onion powder
½ tsp dried oregano, ground
¼ tsp sea salt
¼ tsp smoked paprika

For linguine pasta:

8 oz linguine pasta
1 tsp butter
¼ tsp salt
¼ tsp dried thyme

Directions:

1. Combine soy sauce, chicken broth, garlic powder, onion powder, oregano, salt, and smoked paprika in a small mixing bowl.
2. Grease the stainless steel insert of your Instant Pot with olive oil. Press Sauté button and heat up. Add chicken and broccoli and cook for 5 minutes, stirring occasionally. Pour in the previously prepared sauce and give it a good stir. Cook for 2 more minutes. Remove to a large bowl and cover with a lid.
3. Now, pour 1 ½ cup of water in the inner pot. Add pasta and sprinkle with some salt and thyme. Securely lock the lid and set the steam release handle by moving the valve to the Sealing position. Press the Manual button and set the timer for 4 minutes. Cook on High pressure.
4. When done, perform a quick pressure release and open the pot. Drain the pasta and remove the liquid.
5. Add the butter to the pot. Using a wooden spatula, stir until melts over a Sauté mode. Return the pasta to the pot and cook for 2 minutes, stirring constantly.
6. Transfer the pasta to a serving plate and top with chicken. Garnish with some basil leaves and serve immediately.

Freestyle Points Per Serving: 4

(Calories 199 | Total Fats 8.7g | Net Carbs: 1.3g | Protein 27.1g |Fiber: 0.6g)

Caesar Salad

 Prep Time: 5 MIN |  Cook Time: 7 MIN |  Serves: 5

Ingredients:

For cooking:

Nonstick cooking spray

For chicken:

1 lb chicken breasts, thinly sliced
Salt
Black pepper

For salad:

1 cup Iceberg lettuce, roughly chopped

For dressing:

¼ cup Greek yogurt, fat-free
2 garlic cloves, crushed
2 tsp mayonnaise, low-fat
1 tbsp white wine vinegar
2 oz Grana Padano cheese, grated

Directions:

1. Combine all dressing ingredients in a medium-sized bowl. Mix until well combined and set aside.
2. Plug in the Instant Pot and spray the stainless steel insert with some nonstick cooking spray. Add chicken breasts and sprinkle with some salt and pepper. Cook for 3-4 minutes on each side. Remove from the pot and set aside.
3. Now, roughly chop the lettuce and place in a large salad bowl. Toss in the chicken and top with previously prepared dressing.
4. Serve immediately.

Freestyle Points Per Serving: 5

(Calories 215 | Total Fats 9.2g | Net Carbs: 1.2g | Protein 30.4g |Fiber: 0.1g)

Mozzarella Tomato Turkey

 Prep Time: 10 MIN |  Cook Time: 10 MIN | 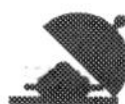 Serves: 4

Ingredients:

For cooking:

Nonstick cooking spray

For turkey:

1 lb turkey breasts, cut into bite-sized pieces
½ tsp dried thyme, ground
¼ tsp dried rosemary, ground
1 tsp tomato paste

For Mozzarella tomato:

1 cup Roma tomatoes, diced
¼ cup Mozzarella cheese
1 tsp dry sherry
2 tsp fresh basil, finely chopped
¼ tsp sea salt

Directions:

1. Rinse the fillets under running water and pat dry with a kitchen paper. Cut into bite-sized pieces and place in a bowl. Add tomato paste, thyme, rosemary, salt, and pepper. Using your hands, mix to coat all. Set aside.
2. Plug in the Instant Pot and spray the stainless steel insert with some nonstick cooking spray. Press the Sauté button and add turkey chops. Cook for 5 minutes, stirring occasionally.
3. Add diced tomatoes, mozzarella, dry sherry, basil, and salt. Stir well and bring it to a boil. Simmer for 5 more minutes.
4. Turn off the pot and transfer all to a serving bowl.
5. Optionally, drizzle with some lemon juice and garnish with some fresh parsley before serving. Enjoy!

Freestyle Points Per Serving: 3

(Calories 136 | Total Fats 2.3g | Net Carbs: 5.7g | Protein 20.3g |Fiber: 1.3g)

Orange Glazed Duck

 Prep Time: 15 MIN |  Cook Time: 15 MIN |  Serves: 4

Ingredients:

For cooking:
1 cup chicken stock, reduced sodium
2 tsp dry sherry

For duck:
1 lb duck breasts, skinless and boneless
1 small red onion, chopped
¼ cup baby carrot, sliced
1 tbsp fresh parsley, finely chopped

Seasoning:
1 tsp fresh thyme, finely chopped
1 tsp fresh rosemary, finely chopped
½ tsp cumin, ground
Salt
Black pepper

For orange sauce:
1 large orange, freshly juiced
1 tsp butter, melted
1 tsp red wine vinegar
1 tsp all-purpose flour
1 tsp sugar

Directions:

1. Plug in the Instant Pot and pour the chicken stock and dry sherry in the stainless steel insert. Add meat and vegetables. Sprinkle with thyme, rosemary, cumin, salt, and pepper. Stir well and pour ½ cup of water in.
2. Securely lock the lid and adjust the steam release handle by turning the valve to the Sealing position. Press the Manual button and set the timer for 8 minutes. Cook on High pressure.
3. Meanwhile, combine all sauce ingredients in a small saucepan over medium-high heat. Stir well and bring it to a boil. Remove from the heat and set aside.
4. When you hear the cooker's end signal, perform a quick pressure release and open the pot.
5. Stir in the orange sauce and press the Sauté button. Cook for 2 more minutes and turn off the pot.
6. Transfer to a serving dish and sprinkle with some finely chopped parsley.

Freestyle Points Per Serving: 3

(Calories 160 | Total Fats 4.7g | Net Carbs: 1.6g | Protein 25.3g |Fiber: 0.4g)

Chicken with Peppers and Peas

 Prep Time: 10 MIN | 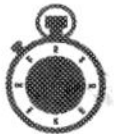 Cook Time: 10 MIN |  Serves: 5

Ingredients:

For cooking:

Nonstick cooking spray

For chicken:

1 lb chicken fillets, skinless, boneless and cut into bite-sized pieces

1 tsp olive oil

½ tsp dried thyme, ground

¼ tsp dried marjoram, ground

Salt

Black pepper

For peas and peppers:

½ cup green peas, frozen

2 large yellow bell pepper, cut into strips

1 small onion, sliced

1 tsp butter

Salt

Directions:

1. Rinse the meat under cold running water and pat dry with a kitchen paper. Transfer to a large cutting board and cut into bite-sized pieces. Set aside.

1. Combine olive oil, thyme, marjoram, salt, and pepper in a small bowl. Mix until combined and drizzle the meat. Mix with your hands until well coated.
2. Grease the stainless steel insert of your Instant Pot with some cooking spray. Press the Sauté button and add chicken. Cook for 4.5 minutes, or until lightly golden brown. Remove from the pot to a bowl and cover with a lid.
3. Now, add butter and gently stir with a wooden spatula until melts. Add onion and bell peppers. Sprinkle with some salt and stir-fry for 2-3 minutes or until softened. Remove from the pot and add peas.
4. Plug in the Instant Pot and pour the chicken stock and dry sherry in the stainless steel insert. Add meat and vegetables. Sprinkle with thyme, rosemary, cumin, salt, and pepper. Stir well and pour ½ cup of water. Securely lock the lid and adjust the steam release handle. Press the Manual button and cook for 3 minutes on High pressure.
5. When done, perform a quick pressure release and open the pot.
6. Serve chicken with bell peppers and peas. Enjoy!

Freestyle Points Per Serving: 5

(Calories 220 | Total Fats 8.6g | Net Carbs: 5.4g | Protein 27.7g |Fiber: 1.7g)

Spicy Turkey Risotto

 Prep Time: 10 MIN |  Cook Time: 10 MIN |  Serves: 6

Ingredients:

For cooking:

Nonstick cooking spray

For turkey risotto:

8 oz turkey breasts, skinless, boneless and cut into bite-sized pieces
1 ½ cup brown rice
3 large egg whites
¼ cup spring onions, finely chopped
1 small carrot, cut into small cubes
1 tbsp soy sauce, reduced sodium

Seasoning:

½ tsp garlic powder
½ tsp turmeric powder
1 tsp chili powder
Salt
Black pepper

Directions:

1. Plug in the Instant Pot and grease the stainless steel insert with some cooking spray. Press the Sauté button and add turkey. Sprinkle with some garlic powder, salt, and pepper. Cook for 5 minutes, or until golden brown.
2. Remove the turkey from the pot and add egg whites. Cook for 2 minutes and then transfer to a bowl with turkey. Cover with a lid and set aside.
3. Now, add rice and carrots to the pot. Sprinkle with turmeric powder, chili powder, and some salt to taste. Stir well and pour in 2 cups of water. Press the Rice mode and set the timer for 7 minutes. Cook on High pressure.
4. When done perform a quick pressure release and open the pot. Stir in the soy sauce and green onions. Press the Sauté button and cook for another 2 minutes.
5. Stir in the egg whites and turn off the pot.
6. Transfer all to a bowl with turkey and give it a good stir to combine. Enjoy!

Freestyle Points Per Serving: 6

(Calories 226 | Total Fats 1.9g | Net Carbs: 37.1g | Protein 12.1g |Fiber: 2.1g)

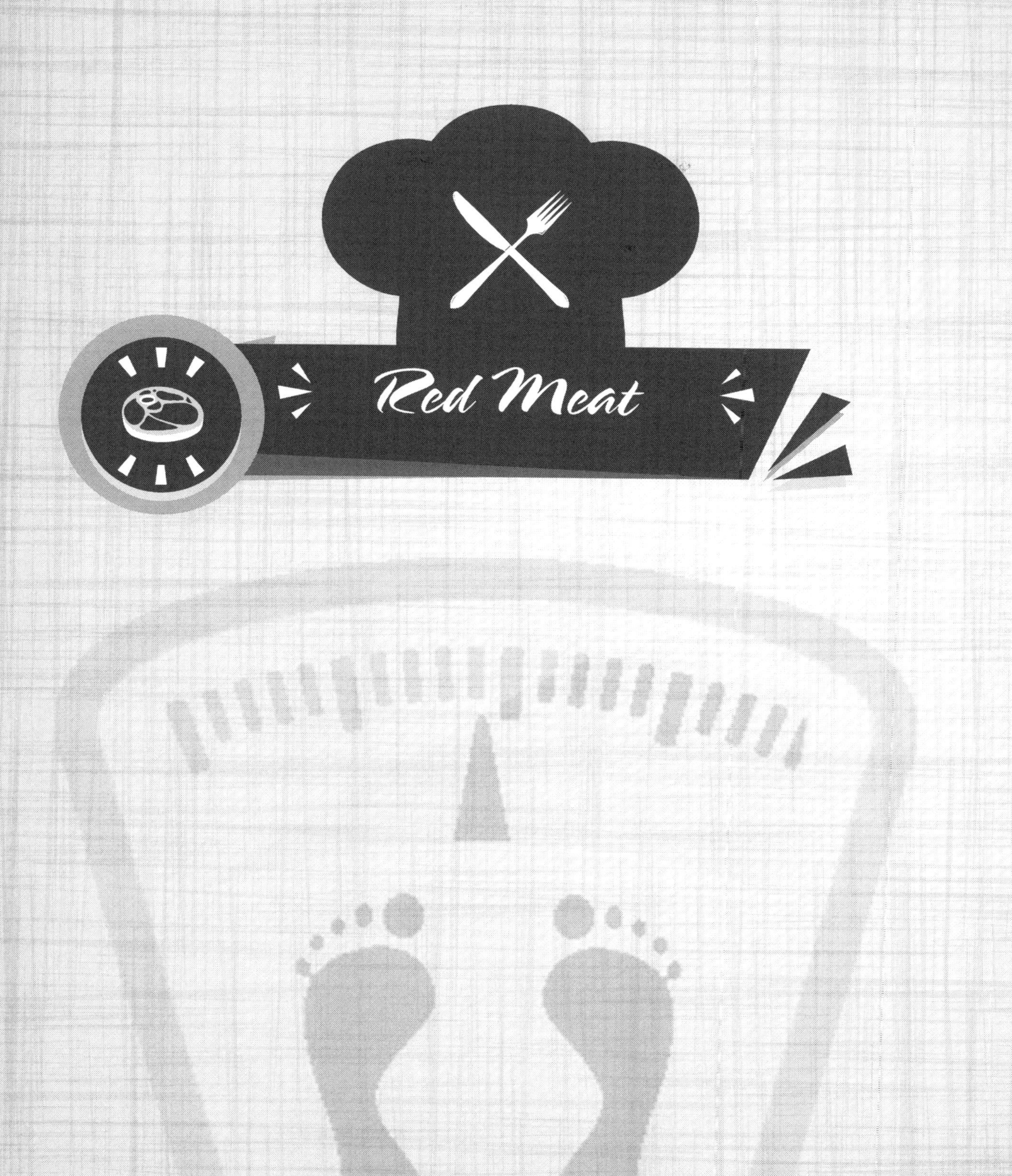
Red Meat

Beef Stir Fry

 Prep Time: 10 MIN |  Cook Time: 5 MIN |  Serves: 4

Ingredients:

For cooking:

1 tbsp olive oil

For stir-fry:

10oz beef sirloin, fat removed
2 yellow bell peppers, sliced
7oz green beans, canned
2 spring onions, chopped
2 tbsp soy sauce

Seasoning:

½ tsp garlic powder
½ tsp salt
¼ tsp black pepper

Directions:

1. Plug in the Instant Pot and press the Sauté button. Grease the inner pot with olive oil and heat up.
2. Place the meat on a cutting board and thinly slice. Add to the pot and cook for 2-3 minutes, stirring constantly.
3. Now add bell peppers, spring onions, and green beans. Sprinkle with soy sauce and season with salt, pepper, and garlic powder.
4. Continue to cook for another 2-3 minutes, stirring constantly.
5. When done, press the Cancel button and serve immediately.

Freestyle Points Per Serving: 5

(Calories 203 | Total Fats 8.1g | Net Carbs: 6.4g | Protein 23.6g |Fiber: 2.8g)

Greek Moussaka

 Prep Time: 15 MIN |  Cook Time: 25 MIN |  Serves: 6

Ingredients:

For cooking:

1 tbsp olive oil

For moussaka:

3 eggplants, sliced
1 lb lean ground beef
1 onion, finely chopped
1 garlic clove, crushed
1 cup tomatoes, diced
1 tbsp tomato puree
2 tbsp Parmesan cheese

Seasoning:

1 tsp salt
½ tsp black pepper
1 tsp dried rosemary

Directions:

1. Slice eggplants lengthwise and sprinkle with some salt. Set aside.
2. Plug in the Instant Pot and press the Sauté button. Grease the inner pot with olive oil and heat up. Add onions and garlic and stir-fry for 3-4 minutes.

1. Now add the meat, diced tomatoes, tomato puree, rosemary, and some salt and pepper to taste. Cook for 6-7 minutes, stirring constantly.
2. Press the Cancel button and remove the meat from the pot. Set aside.
3. Rinse the eggplant slices and gently press with your hands. Spread half of the eggplants over a small fitting casserole dish and add the meat. Top with the remaining eggplant slices and sprinkle with parmesan cheese. Optionally, season with some more salt and pepper to taste. Loosely cover with aluminum foil and set aside.
4. Now, set the trivet at the bottom of the inner pot and pour in one cup of water. Place the casserole dish on top and seal the lid.
5. Set the steam release handle to the Sealing position and press the Manual button.
6. Set the timer for 13 minutes on High pressure.
7. When done, perform a quick pressure release and open the lid. Remove the dish from the pot and cool for a while.
8. Slice and serve.

Freestyle Points Per Serving: 7

(Calories 251 | Total Fats 8.1g | Net Carbs: 9g | Protein 26.9g |Fiber: 10.5g)

Beef Steak with Herbs

 Prep Time: 10 MIN |  Cook Time: 10 MIN |  Serves: 2

Ingredients:

For cooking:

1 tbsp oil

For beef steak:

2 beef steaks, about 3.5oz each
2 tbsp freshly squeezed lemon juice
1 garlic clove, crushed

Seasoning:

½ tsp garlic salt
1 tsp dried thyme
½ tsp dried basil
¼ tsp white pepper

Directions:

1. Plug in the Instant Pot and press the Sauté button.
2. Rub each steak with oil and generously sprinkle with garlic salt, thyme, basil, and pepper.
3. Place in the pot and cook for 5 minutes on each side.
4. When done, press the Cancel button and remove the steaks from the pot.
5. Serve immediately.

Freestyle Points Per Serving: 5

(Calories 250 | Total Fats 13.1g | Net Carbs: 0.7g | Protein 30.3g |Fiber: 0.1g)

Easy Beef Stew with Spring Onions

 Prep Time: 15 MIN |  Cook Time: 30 MIN |  Serves: 4

Ingredients:

For cooking:

2 tsp oil
4 cups beef broth, low-sodium

For stew:

1lb lean beef stew meat
2 cups tomatoes, diced
2 spring onions, chopped
2 onions, sliced
2 tbsp fresh parsley, finely chopped

Seasoning:

1 tsp garlic powder
1 tbsp cayenne pepper
1 ½ tsp dried thyme
Salt and pepper to taste

Directions:

1. Place the meat in a deep bowl and sprinkle with salt and pepper.
2. Plug in the Instant Pot and press the Sauté button. Grease the inner pot with oil and heat up.
3. Add the meat and briefly brown for 3-4 minutes, stirring constantly.
4. Stir in tomatoes, onions, and parsley. Continue to cook for 3-4 minutes, stirring constantly.
5. Now, pour in the broth and season with garlic powder, cayenne pepper, and thyme. Seal the lid and press the Stew button.
6. Cook for 20 minutes on high pressure.
7. When done, release the pressure naturally and open the lid. Serve immediately.

Freestyle Points Per Serving: 4

(Calories 174 | Total Fats 5.5g | Net Carbs: 23.8g | Protein 20.4g |Fiber: 2.5g)

Pork Neck with Carrots

 Prep Time: 15 MIN | 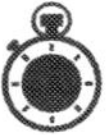 Cook Time: 25 MIN | 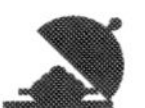 Serves: 4

Ingredients:

For cooking:

1 tbsp oil

3 cups beef stock, low-sodium

For pork:

10oz pork neck, fat removed

2 carrots, sliced

1 medium-sized sweet potato, chopped

1 onion, finely chopped

Seasoning:

1 tbsp dried parsley

2 bay leaves

½ tsp salt

¼ tsp black pepper

Directions:

1. Rinse the meat under cold running water and place on a cutting board. Using a sharp knife, remove fat and chop into bite-sized pieces.
2. Plug in the Instant Pot and grease the inner pot with oil. Heat up and add chopped onion and meat. Season with salt and pepper.
3. Cook for 6-7 minutes, stirring constantly.
4. Now add carrots and sweet potato. Give it a good stir and press the Cancel button.
5. Sprinkle with parsley and add bay leaves. Pour in the stock and stir well.
6. Seal the lid and set the steam release handle to the Sealing position. Press the Manual button and set the timer for 20 minutes on High pressure.
7. When done, release the pressure naturally and carefully open the lid. Cool for a while and serve.

Freestyle Points Per Serving: 6

(Calories 221 | Total Fats 7.7g | Net Carbs: 10.7g | Protein 24g |Fiber: 2.3g)

Beef Steak Salad

 Prep Time: 10 MIN | 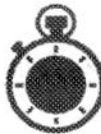 Cook Time: 10 MIN |  Serves: 4

Ingredients:

For cooking:

2 tsp olive oil

For salad:

7oz beef steaks, about 2 pieces
7oz asparagus
1 cup lettuce, torn
1 cup cherry tomatoes, sliced
1 lemon, sliced
2 tbsp lemon juice

Seasoning:

1 tsp dried thyme
½ tsp dried rosemary
½ tsp smoked salt
¼ tsp black pepper, freshly ground

Directions:

1. Plug in the Instant Pot and press the Sauté button. Grease the inner pot with oil and heat up.
2. Meanwhile, rinse the steaks and rub with thyme, rosemary, smoked salt, and pepper. Place in the pot and cook for 4-5 minutes.
3. Meanwhile, rinse and chop asparagus into bite-sized pieces. Add to the pot and stir well.
4. Flip the steaks and continue to cook for another 4-5 minutes.
5. Press the Cancel button and transfer the meat along with asparagus to a deep serving bowl. Cool for a while and slice the steaks. Set aside.
6. Rinse and prepare the vegetables. Place in a bowl and sprinkle with lemon juice. Top with sliced lemon and serve.

Freestyle Points Per Serving: 3

(Calories 138 | Total Fats 5.7g | Net Carbs: 3.5g | Protein 16.8g |Fiber: 2.1g)

Spicy Lamb Shank

 Prep Time: 15 MIN |  Cook Time: 10 MIN |  Serves: 8

Ingredients:

For cooking:

1 tbsp olive oil

For lamb:

10oz lamb shank, fat removed
1 purple onion, chopped
5 garlic cloves, sliced
5 chili peppers, whole
1 cup lettuce, torn
2 tbsp fish sauce
¼ cup lime juice

Seasoning:

½ tsp chili powder
¼ tsp black pepper

Directions:

1. Slice the meat into about 1-inch thick slices and sprinkle with chili powder and pepper. Set aside.
2. Plug in the Instant Pot and heat up the oil. Add onions and cook for 2 minutes.
3. Now add chili peppers and garlic. Cook for 3-4 minutes, stirring constantly. If necessary, pour in about 2 tbsp water.
4. Finally, add the meat and sprinkle with fish sauce. Give it a good stir and optionally season with some more salt or chili powder.
5. Cook for 4-5 minutes, stirring constantly.
6. Press the Cancel button and remove from the pot. Transfer to a bowl and add lettuce.
7. Toss well to combine, drizzle with freshly squeezed lime juice and serve.

Freestyle Points Per Serving: 5

(Calories 209 | Total Fats 7.1g | Net Carbs: 6g | Protein 28.1g |Fiber: 1.3g)

Sweet Cranberry Pork

 Prep Time: 10 MIN | 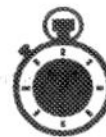 Cook Time: 10 MIN | 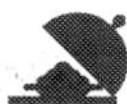 Serves: 3

Ingredients:

For cooking:

1 tbsp coconut oil

For pork:

7oz pork leg, fat removed and sliced
2 cups arugula
1 cup cranberries
2 tbsp pine nuts
1 tbsp lemon juice

Seasoning:

1 tsp coconut sugar
¼ tsp nutmeg

Directions:

1. Place cranberries in the pot and pour in enough water to cover. Stir in coconut sugar and nutmeg.
2. Seal the lid and set the steam release handle to the Sealing position. Press the Manual button and set the timer for 3 minutes on High pressure.
3. When done, release the pressure naturally and open the lid. Transfer to a deep bowl and set aside.
4. Now press the Sauté button and melt the coconut oil. Add pine nuts and cook for 2 minutes.
5. Now add the meat and continue to cook for 5-6 minutes, stirring constantly.
6. Stir in the cranberry sauce and bring it to a boil. Press the Cancel button and remove from the pot.
7. Divide the meat between serving bowls and add arugula. Drizzle with lemon juice and stir well.
8. Serve immediately.

Freestyle Points Per Serving: 6

(Calories 202 | Total Fats 10.9g | Net Carbs: 4.2g | Protein 18.5g |Fiber: 1.8g)

Sriracha Beef Ribs

 Prep Time: 15 MIN |  Cook Time: 35 MIN |  Serves: 8

Ingredients:

For cooking:

1 tbsp oil

For beef:

2 lbs beef ribs
2 onions, chopped
3 garlic cloves, crushed
1 cup tomato sauce, sugar-free
4 tbsp sriracha sauce
3 tbsp fish sauce
2 tbsp lime juice

Seasoning:

½ tsp cumin powder
Salt and pepper to taste

Directions:

1. Place ribs in the pot and pour in about 3 cups of water. Sprinkle with some salt and seal the lid.
2. Set the steam release handle to the Sealing position and press the Manual button. Set the timer for 25 minutes on High pressure.
3. When done, perform a quick pressure release and open the lid. Remove the ribs from the pot and chill for a while.
4. Now press the Sauté button and heat the oil.
5. Add onions and garlic. Give it a good stir and cook for 3-4 minutes.
6. Now add the tomato sauce, sriracha, fish sauce, lime juice, and cumin powder. Season with some more salt and pepper to taste and cook for 2 minutes.
7. Add the meat and coat well with the sauce.
8. Press the Cancel button and serve.

Freestyle Points Per Serving: 5

(Calories 251 | Total Fats 8.9g | Net Carbs: 4.3g | Protein 35.5g |Fiber: 1.1g)

Veal Steaks with Eggplants and Mushrooms

 Prep Time: 10 MIN | 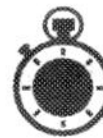 Cook Time: 10 MIN | 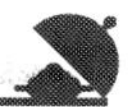 Serves: 4

Ingredients:

For cooking:
1 tbsp oil

For the steaks:
1lb boneless veal steaks, fat removed
1 cucumber, chopped
½ eggplant, sliced
1 cup button mushrooms
½ purple onion, sliced
2 tbsp soy sauce
1 tbsp mirin

Seasoning:
½ tsp salt
¼ tsp black pepper
¼ tsp dried thyme

Directions:

1. Rinse the meat under cold running water and place on a cutting board. Trim any excess fat and chop into bite-sized pieces. Transfer to a bowl and season with salt, pepper, and thyme. Sprinkle with soy sauce and mix well. Set aside.
2. Plug in the Instant Pot and press the Sauté button. Grease the inner pot with oil and add onions. Cook for 2-3 minutes and then add eggplants. Continue to cook for another 2-3 minutes.
3. Finally, add the meat and mushrooms. Sprinkle with mirin and cook for 5-6 minutes.
4. Press the Cancel button and remove from the pot. Mix with cucumber and serve.

Freestyle Points Per Serving: 6

(Calories 257 | Total Fats 10.9g | Net Carbs: 7.4g | Protein 29.6g | Fiber: 2.9g)

Spicy Beef Neck

 Prep Time: 20 MIN |  Cook Time: 30 MIN |  Serves: 4

Ingredients:

For cooking:

1 cup beef stock, low-sodium

For soup:

10oz beef neck, fat removed and chopped into bite-sized pieces
1 cup coconut milk, reduced-fat
2 green bell peppers, sliced
1 small zucchini, sliced
1 chili pepper, whole
¼ cup fish sauce
2 tbsp chili paste

Seasoning:

1 tbsp fresh ginger, grated
2 tbsp fresh parsley, finely chopped

Directions:

1. Plug in the Instant Pot and add the meat. Pour in beef stock and add chili pepper, ginger, and parsley.
2. Seal the lid and set the steam release handle to the Sealing position. Press the Manual button and cook for 20 minutes on the Manual mode.
3. When done, perform a quick pressure release and open the lid. Press the Sauté button and stir in the chili paste and fish sauce. Add zucchini and sliced bell peppers.
4. Cook for 10 minutes, stirring occasionally.
5. Finally, pour in the coconut milk and heat up. Press the Cancel button and serve.

Freestyle Points Per Serving: 6

(Calories 209 | Total Fats 7.8g | Net Carbs: 8.8g | Protein 24.6g |Fiber: 1.2g)

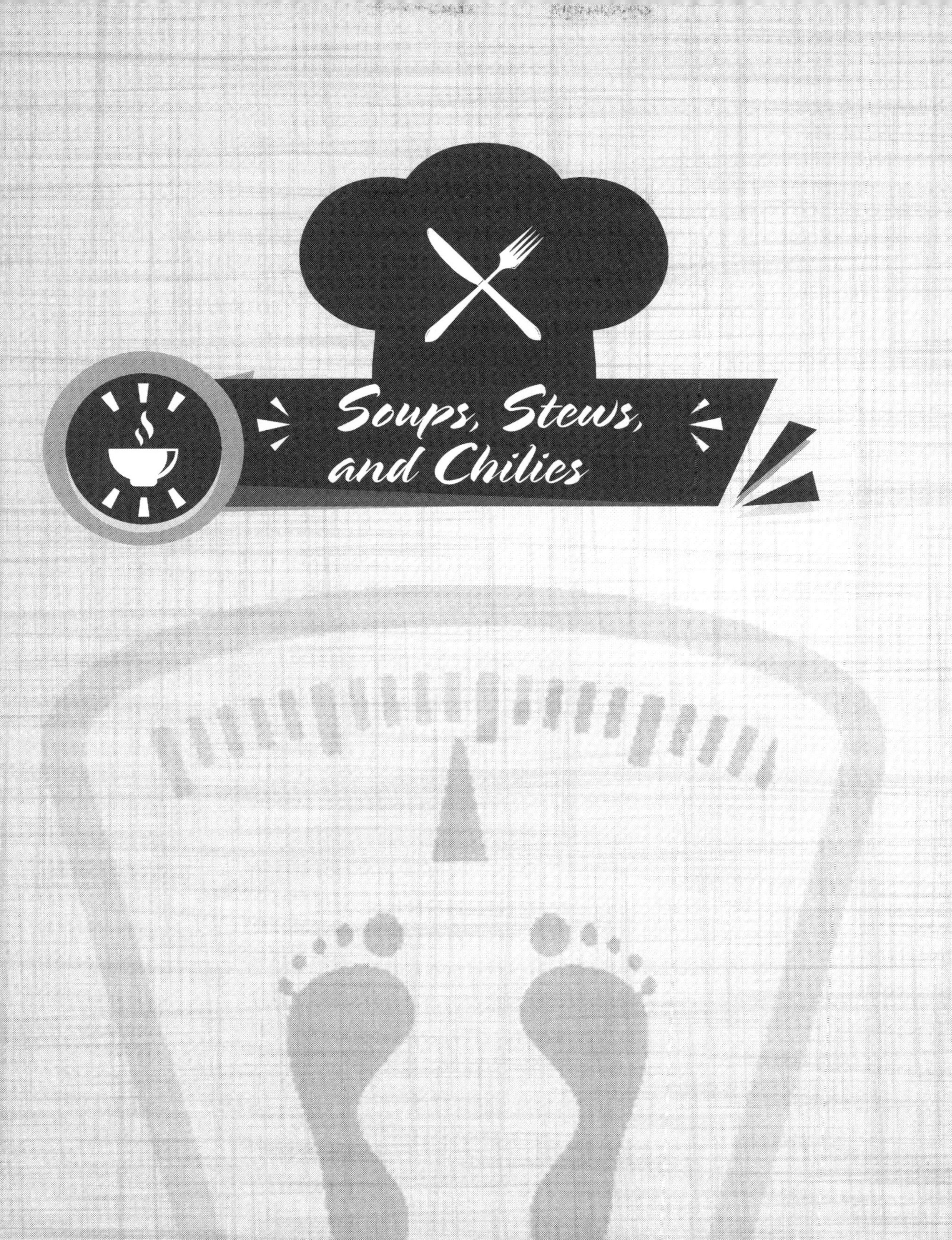

Soups, Stews, and Chilies

Green Chicken Curry

 Prep Time: 15 MIN |  Cook Time: 25 MIN |  Serves: 6

Ingredients:

For cooking:

1 tbsp oil

For curry:

7oz chicken breast
2 tbsp green curry paste
¾ cup coconut milk, reduced fat
½ cup green bell peppers, sliced
2 large onions, finely chopped
1 small tomato, sliced
¼ cup fish sauce

Seasoning:

1 tsp coconut sugar
1 tsp dried basil

Directions:

1. Grease the bottom of the inner pot with oil and heat up on the Sauté mode. Add the meat and briefly cook for 2-3 minutes, stirring constantly.
2. Now add green bell peppers, onions, and tomato. Cook for another 3-4 minutes, stirring constantly.
3. Pour in the coconut milk and 2 cups of water. Add green curry paste and bring it to a boil, stirring constantly.
4. Add the remaining ingredients and seal the lid. Set the steam release handle and cook for 20 minutes on the Manual mode.
5. When done, perform a quick pressure release and open the lid. Serve immediately.

Freestyle Points Per Serving: 5

(Calories 174 | Total Fats 11.4g | Net Carbs: 8g | Protein 9.1g |Fiber: 2g)

Chili con Carne

 Prep Time: 15 MIN |  Cook Time: 30 MIN |  Serves: 8

Ingredients:

For cooking:

1 tbsp oil

For curry:

10oz lean ground beef
2 small onions, finely chopped
2 garlic cloves, crushed
1 cup tomatoes, diced
¼ cup red kidney beans
¼ cup canned corn
2 small chili peppers, diced

Seasoning:

2 tsp chili powder
¼ tsp salt
½ tsp cumin powder
½ tsp dried oregano
¼ tsp red pepper sauce

Directions:

1. Plug in the Instant Pot and press the Sauté button. Heat up the oil and add onions, garlic, chili pepper, and ground beef. Cook for 3-4 minutes, stirring constantly.
2. Stir in the remaining ingredients and pour in 3 cups of water.
3. Seal the lid and set the steam release handle to the Sealing position.
4. Cook for 20 minutes on the Stew mode.
5. When done, release the pressure naturally and open the lid.
6. Serve immediately.

Freestyle Points Per Serving: 6

(Calories 234 | Total Fats 8.2g | Net Carbs: 11.2g | Protein 25.3g |Fiber: 3.4g)

Chicken Stew with Onions

 Prep Time: 15 MIN |  Cook Time: 30+5 MIN |  Serves: 8

Ingredients:

For cooking:

1 tbsp oil
4 cups chicken stock, low-sodium

For curry:

10oz chicken breast, chopped into bite-sized pieces
4 onions, chopped
3 garlic cloves, crushed
1 cup tomatoes, diced

Seasoning:

1 tsp turmeric powder
2 tsp fennel seeds
½ tsp cumin powder
1 tbsp cayenne pepper
½ tsp salt

Directions:

1. Place onions with all spices in a food processor and process until a smooth paste. Set aside.
2. Heat the oil on the Sauté mode and add fennel seeds. Cook for 1 minute.
3. Stir in onions and cook for another minute.
4. Then add the chicken and brown for 4-5 minutes on all sides. Stir all well and add garlic cloves and tomatoes.
5. Pour in ¼ cup water and continue to cook for 10-12 minutes.
6. Finally, pour in the stock and seal the lid. Set the steam release handle and cook for 20 minutes on the Manual mode.
7. When done, perform a quick pressure release and open the lid.
8. Serve immediately.

Freestyle Points Per Serving: 5

(Calories 176 | Total Fats 5.9g | Net Carbs: 10.5g | Protein 17.5g |Fiber: 3g)

Buckwheat Veal Stew

 Prep Time: 15 MIN |  Cook Time: 40 MIN |  Serves: 4

Ingredients:

For cooking:

1 tbsp oil

3 cups beef stock, low-sodium

For curry:

7oz veal shoulder, chopped into bite-sized pieces

¼ cup buckwheat groats

2 carrots, sliced

1 onion, chopped

1 tomato, chopped

2 tbsp lemon juice

Seasoning:

Salt and pepper to taste

2 bay leaves

2 tbsp parsley, finely chopped

Directions:

1. Plug in the Instant Pot and add groats. Pour in enough water to cover and seal the lid. Cook for 3 minutes on the Manual mode.
2. When done, perform a quick pressure release and open the lid. Drain the buckwheat and set aside.
3. Now press the Sauté button. Heat up the oil and add onions. Season with some salt and cook for 3-4 minutes.
4. Add the meat, tomato, and carrots. Season with the remaining salt and continue to cook for 5 minutes, stirring constantly.
5. Add the remaining ingredients and pour in the stock. Sprinkle with lemon juice and seal the lid.
6. Set the steam release handle to the Sealing position and press the Manual mode.
7. Set the timer for 30 minutes on High pressure.
8. When done, release the pressure naturally and open the lid. Serve immediately.

Freestyle Points Per Serving: 4

(Calories 187 | Total Fats 7.8g | Net Carbs: 9.4g | Protein 17.4g |Fiber: 2.3g)

Chicken Soup with Mushrooms

 Prep Time: 30 MIN |  Cook Time: 20 MIN |  Serves: 6

Ingredients:

For cooking:

4 cups chicken stock, low-sodium
1 tbsp olive oil

For curry:

7oz chicken breast, chopped into bite-sized pieces
1 onion, finely chopped
3 garlic cloves, crushed
3 carrots, sliced
2 tbsp celery roots, chopped
2 cups button mushrooms, sliced
2 tbsp all-purpose flour
½ cup heavy cream

Seasoning:

Salt and pepper to taste
2 bay leaves
2 tbsp fresh parsley, finely chopped

Directions:

1. Rinse the meat thoroughly and pat dry with a kitchen towel. Chop into bite-sized pieces and set aside.
2. Plug in the Instant Pot and press the Sauté button. Grease the inner pot with olive oil and heat up. Add chopped chicken and briefly brown for 3-4 minutes, stirring constantly.
3. Now add garlic, carrots, celery, and chopped onion. Continue to cook for 2-3 minutes.
4. Press the Cancel button and add mushrooms. Pour in the stock and season with salt and pepper to taste.
5. Add bay leaves and sprinkle with fresh parsley. Stir all well and seal the lid.
6. Set the steam release handle to the Sealing position and press the Manual button.
7. Cook for 15 minutes on High pressure.
8. When done, perform a quick pressure release and open the lid. Stir in flour and heavy cream.
9. Let it sit, covered, for 10-15 minutes before serving.

Freestyle Points Per Serving: 4

(Calories 136 | Total Fats 7.4g | Net Carbs: 7.5g | Protein 9.3g |Fiber: 1.5g)

Italian Green Beans Stew

 Prep Time: 10 MIN |  Cook Time: 20 MIN |  Serves: 4

Ingredients:

For cooking:

2 cups chicken stock, low-sodium
1 tbsp oil

For curry:

1 lb green beans
2 large tomatoes, roughly chopped
1 large onion, finely chopped
2 tbsp tomato puree
2 tbsp Parmesan, grated

Seasoning:

2 tsp cayenne pepper
½ tsp chili powder
2 rosemary sprigs, fresh
Salt and pepper to taste

Directions:

1. Heat the oil on the Sauté mode and add onions. Stir well and cook for 2-3 minutes.
2. Now add tomatoes and stir in tomato puree. Continue to cook for 3-4 minutes.
3. Finally, add beans and season with salt, pepper, chili powder, and cayenne pepper. Add rosemary sprigs and pour in the stock.
4. Seal the lid and set the steam release handle to the Sealing position.
5. Cook for 15 minutes on the Manual mode.
6. When done, perform a quick pressure release and open the lid. Sprinkle with grated Parmesan and serve.

Freestyle Points Per Serving: 4

(Calories 125 | Total Fats 5.5g | Net Carbs: 10.1g | Protein 5.9g |Fiber: 5.8g)

Veal Stew with Kale

 Prep Time: 20 MIN |  Cook Time: 35 MIN |  Serves: 6

Ingredients:

For cooking:

4 cups beef stock, low sodium

For curry:

10oz veal shoulder, fat removed
2 large onions, finely chopped
3 carrots, sliced
1 lb fresh kale, chopped
1 small sweet potato, diced
3 garlic cloves, crushed
2 celery stalks, chopped

Seasoning:

½ tsp salt
1 tsp onion powder
½ tsp dried basil

Directions:

1. Plug in the Instant Pot and press the Sauté button. Grease the inner pot with oil and add onions and garlic. Cook for 3-4 minutes, or until translucent.
2. Now add carrots, celery stalk, and chopped sweet potato. Pour in ¼ cup of stock and season with salt, onion powder, and basil. Give it a good stir and cook for 5 minutes.
3. Meanwhile, rinse the meat under cold running water and place on a cutting board. Remove any visible fat and chop into bite-sized pieces.
4. Add to the pot along with chopped kale.
5. Pour in the remaining stock and seal the lid. Set the steam release handle to the Sealing position and press the Manual button.
6. Cook for 25 minutes on high pressure.
7. When done, release the pressure naturally and open the lid.
8. Serve immediately.

Freestyle Points Per Serving: 5

(Calories 214 | Total Fats 5.3g | Net Carbs: 15g | Protein 23.5g |Fiber: 3.4g)

Mushroom Goulash

 Prep Time: 20 MIN |  Cook Time: 40 MIN |  Serves: 6

Ingredients:

For cooking:

3 cups beef stock, low sodium

For curry:

1 lb beef ribs, fat removed
2 cups button mushrooms, sliced
1 bacon slice, chopped
2 celery stalks, chopped
2 large carrots, sliced
¼ cup sour cream

Seasoning:

½ tsp salt
1 bay leaf
1 tsp dried basil
1 tsp peppercorn
1 tbsp cayenne pepper

Directions:

1. Season the meat with salt and place in the pot. Pour in the stock and seal the lid.
1. Cook for 30 minutes on the Manual mode. When done, release the pressure naturally and open the lid.
1. Remove the meat from the pot and place on a cutting board. Using a sharp knife, remove the bones and place the meat back into the pot.
1. Stir in mushrooms, chopped bacon, celery stalks, and carrots. Add bay leaf, basil, peppercorn, and cayenne pepper.
1. Set the steam release handle to the Sealing position and press the Manual button.
1. Cook for 7 minutes on High pressure.
1. When done, perform a quick pressure release and open the lid.
1. Stir in the sour cream and serve.

Freestyle Points Per Serving: 5

(Calories 202 | Total Fats 8.4g | Net Carbs: 2.9g | Protein 26.7g |Fiber: 0.9g)

Spring Fish Soup

 Prep Time: 10 MIN |  Cook Time: 25 MIN |  Serves: 8

Ingredients:

For cooking:

1 tbsp olive oil

3 cups fish stock, low-sodium

For curry:

1 lb trout fillets

¼ cup brown rice

2 carrots, sliced

2 onions, sliced

3 garlic cloves

¼ cup white wine

2 tbsp celery root, chopped

Seasoning:

Salt and pepper to taste

½ tsp rosemary powder

½ tsp garlic powder

1 bay leaf

Directions:

1. Chop the fillets into bite-sized pieces and sprinkle with salt and pepper. Set aside.
2. Heat up the oil and add garlic and celery root. Cook for 1 minute and then add onions. Season with rosemary and garlic powder.
3. Cook for 3-4 minutes.
4. Now add the fillets and stir well. Cook for 2-3 minutes.
5. Finally, add the remaining ingredients and pour in the stock. Stir all well and seal the lid.
6. Set the steam release handle to the Sealing position and press the Stew button. Set the timer for 15 minutes on High pressure.
7. When done, perform a quick pressure release and open the lid. Remove the bay leaf and serve.

Freestyle Points Per Serving: 4

(Calories 185 | Total Fats 7.5g | Net Carbs: 8.2g | Protein 18.1g |Fiber: 1.2g)

Beef and Pork Stew

 Prep Time: 15 MIN |  Cook Time: 8 HOURS 5 MIN |  Serves: 8

Ingredients:

For cooking:

1 tbsp oil

4 cups beef stock, low-sodium

For curry:

1 lb lean ground beef

10oz pork shoulder, chopped into bite-sized pieces

2 carrots, sliced

¼ cup parsley, finely chopped

3 garlic cloves, crushed

2 onions, chopped

2 cups tomato sauce, sugar-free

2 tbsp apple cider vinegar

Seasoning:

Salt and pepper to taste

2 bay leaves

1 tbsp cayenne pepper

Directions:

1. Plug in the Instant Pot and press the Sauté button. Grease the inner pot with oil and heat up. Add onions, garlic, and chopped pork. Cook for 3-4 minutes, stirring constantly.
2. Then add the beef and continue to cook for another minute.
3. Season with some salt and pepper to taste and add bay leaves. Sprinkle with cayenne pepper and add the remaining ingredients. Pour in the stock and seal the lid.
4. Set the steam release handle to the Sealing position and press the Slow Cooker button.
5. Set the timer for 8 hours on Low pressure.
6. When done, release the pressure naturally and remove the bay leaves.
7. Serve immediately.

Freestyle Points Per Serving: 5

(Calories 230 | Total Fats 8.7g | Net Carbs: 5.9g | Protein 29.1g |Fiber: 2g)

Cheese and Wine Soup

 Prep Time: 10 MIN |  Cook Time: 10 MIN |  Serves: 4

Ingredients:

For cooking:

1 tbsp oil
3 cups chicken stock

For curry:

¼ cup white wine
¼ cup gorgonzola cheese, crumbled
¼ cup Gouda cheese, grated
½ cup heavy cream, reduced fat
2 tbsp plain Greek yogurt, fat-free
2 slices whole grain bread, chopped into bite-sized pieces

Seasoning:

Salt and white pepper to taste
1 tbsp fresh chives, chopped

Directions:

1. Plug in the Instant Pot and press the Sauté button. Grease the inner pot with oil and heat up. Add gorgonzola cheese and gently melt, stirring constantly.
2. Stir in the Greek yogurt and pour in the heavy cream. Add bread and cook for 2-3 minutes, stirring constantly.
3. Now add the wine and sprinkle with Gouda cheese. Season with salt, pepper, and chopped chives. Give it a good stir and pour in the stock.
4. Seal the lid and set the steam release handle to the Sealing position. Cook for 3 minutes on the Manual mode.
5. When done, release the pressure naturally and open the lid.
6. Serve immediately.

Freestyle Points Per Serving: 5

(Calories 135 | Total Fats 7.9g | Net Carbs: 8.1g | Protein 5.3g |Fiber: 1.3g)

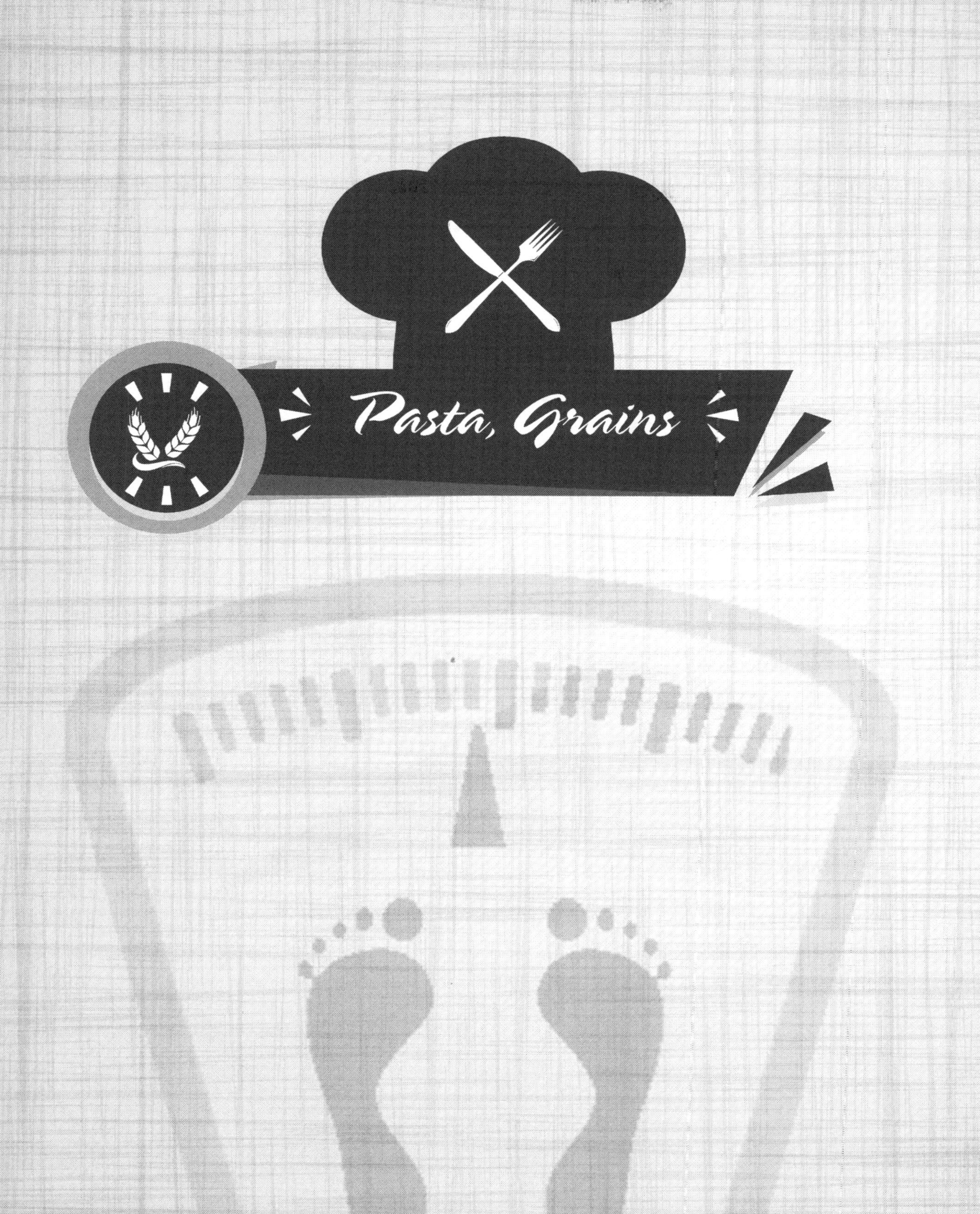
Pasta, Grains

Cheesy Rigatoni

 Prep Time: 10 MIN |  Cook Time: 17 MIN |  Serves: 7

Ingredients:

For cooking:

1 tsp butter

For rigatoni:

10 oz rigatoni pasta
8 oz broccoli, chopped
1 cup cheddar cheese, grated
½ cup heavy cream
1 cup tomatoes, diced
1 small onion, diced
1 tsp fresh lemon juice

Seasoning:

½ tsp dried oregano, ground
1 tsp sugar
1 tsp Italian seasoning
½ tsp red pepper flakes
Salt

Directions:

1. Place the pasta in the stainless steel insert of your Instant Pot. Sprinkle with some salt and securely lock the lid. Set the steam release handle and press the Manual button. Set the timer for 7 minutes and cook on High pressure.
2. When done, perform a quick pressure release and open the pot. Using a large colander, drain the pasta and remove the water.
3. Press the Sauté button and add butter. Gently stir until butter has completely melted. Add broccoli, onions, and heavy cream. Bring it to a boil and simmer for 3-4 minutes.
4. Add tomatoes, lemon juice, sugar, oregano, Italian seasoning, and red pepper flakes. Stir well and simmer for 6-7 minutes.
5. Finally, add pasta and give it a good stir.
6. Optionally, garnish with some fresh basil leaves and serve immediately.

Freestyle Points Per Serving: 7

(Calories 216 | Total Fats 10g | Net Carbs: 22.6g | Protein 8.8g |Fiber: 0g)

Brown Rice with Peppers

 Prep Time: 5 MIN |  Cook Time: 5 MIN | 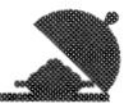 Serves: 7

Ingredients:

For cooking:

1 tsp olive oil

For rice:

2 cups brown rice
1 red bell pepper, chopped
1 yellow bell pepper, chopped
½ cup green peas
1 small carrot, cut into small cubes
1 tsp fish sauce
1 tsp soy sauce

Seasoning:

½ tsp turmeric powder
½ tsp onion powder
¼ tsp dried rosemary, ground
1 small saffron thread

Directions:

1. Plug in the Instant Pot and press the Sauté button. Add bell peppers and stir-fry for 5 minutes.
2. Add rice, green peas, and carrots. Pour in the fish sauce and soy sauce. Stir well and add 3 cups of water. Securely lock the lid and adjust the steam release handle. Press the Manual button and set the timer for 4 minutes. Cook on High pressure.
3. When you hear the cooker's end signal, perform a quick pressure release and open the pot.
4. Stir in the turmeric powder, onion powder, rosemary, and saffron. Press the Sauté button and cook for 1 minute.
5. Transfer to a serving plate and garnish with some fresh parsley before serving. Enjoy!

Freestyle Points Per Serving: 7

(Calories 225 | Total Fats 2.2g | Net Carbs: 43.2g | Protein 5.1g |Fiber: 3g)

Cauliflower Vermicelli

 Prep Time: 10 MIN |  Cook Time: 20 MIN |  Serves:

Ingredients:

For cooking:

1 tsp olive oil

For vermicelli:

1 cup cauliflower, chopped
12 oz vermicelli pasta
1 small green chili pepper, chopped
1 cup tomatoes, diced
1 tsp fresh lime juice
2 tbsp green onions, chopped
1 tsp mirin
1 tsp soy sauce
2 tbsp fresh parsley, finely chopped

Seasoning:

1 tsp dried oregano, ground
1 tsp smoked paprika, ground
Salt
Black pepper

Directions:

1. Plug in the Instant Pot, add pasta and enough water to cover and sprinkle with some salt. Securely lock the lid and adjust the steam release handle. Press the Manual button and cook on High pressure for 7 minutes.
2. When done, perform a quick release of the pressure and open the pot. Drain the pasta and transfer to a large bowl. Cover with a lid and set aside.
3. Remove the water from the pot and pat dry with kitchen paper.
4. Now, heat up the olive oil over a Sauté mode. Add cauliflower and chili pepper. Cook for 5 minutes, stirring occasionally. Add mirin, soy sauce, lime juice, and parsley. Sprinkle with oregano, paprika, and salt. Cook for 2 more minutes and then add tomatoes. Stir well and bring it to a boil. Cook for 5 more minutes and turn off the pot.
5. Stir in the pasta and transfer all to a serving dish. Sprinkle with green onions before serving and enjoy!

Freestyle Points Per Serving: 5

(Calories 199 | Total Fats 1.6g | Net Carbs: 36.3g | Protein 6.7g |Fiber: 2.5g)

Quick Spicy Couscous

 Prep Time: 5 MIN |  Cook Time: 3 MIN | 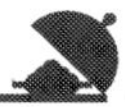 Serves: 5

Ingredients:

For cooking:

1 tsp olive oil
4 cups chicken broth, reduced sodium

For couscous:

2 cups couscous
1 small onion, diced
1 small carrot, diced
¼ cup fresh parsley, finely chopped

Seasoning:

½ tsp chili powder
¼ tsp garlic powder
½ tsp sea salt
¼ tsp black pepper, ground

Directions:

1. Place the butter in your Instant Pot. Press the Sauté button and gently stir until the butter has completely melted.
2. Add onions and sprinkle with garlic powder. Cook for 2-3 minutes, or until soft.
3. Add couscous and carrot. Sprinkle with chili powder, salt, and pepper. Stir well and pour in the chicken stock.
4. Securely lock the lid and adjust the steam release handle. Press the Manual button and set the timer for 3 minutes. Cook on High pressure.
5. When you hear the cooker's end signal, perform a quick pressure release by moving the valve to the Venting position.
6. Open the pot and stir in the parsley. Transfer to a serving dish and serve immediately. Enjoy!

Freestyle Points Per Serving: 8

(Calories 310 | Total Fats 2.5g | Net Carbs: 52.7g | Protein 13g |Fiber: 4.1g)

Turkey Risotto

 Prep Time: 10 MIN |  Cook Time: 13 MIN | 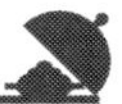 Serves: 4

Ingredients:

For cooking:
1 tsp olive oil

For risotto:
2 cups white rice
4 oz chicken breasts, skinless and boneless
½ cup green peas
¼ cup fresh cilantro, chopped
1 medium-sized red bell pepper, chopped
1 small onion, chopped
2 garlic cloves, minced

Seasoning:
½ tsp turmeric powder
½ tsp red pepper
½ tsp dried basil, ground
Salt

Directions:

1. Rinse the meat under cold running water and pat dry with a kitchen paper. Transfer to a cutting board and cut into bite-sized pieces. Set aside.
2. Plug in the Instant Pot and add olive oil to the stainless steel insert. Press the Sauté button and heat. Add turkey chops and sprinkle with some salt and pepper. Cook for 4-5 minutes, or until golden brown. Remove from the pot to a bowl and cover with a lid. Set aside.
3. Add onions, garlic, and bell pepper. Stir-fry for 3-4 minutes, or until the onions translucent. Add rice and green peas. Pour in 2 cups of water. Securely lock the lid and adjust the steam release handle.
4. Set the Manual mode and cook for 4 minutes on High pressure.
5. When you hear the cooker's end signal, perform a quick pressure release. Open the pot and stir in the previously cooked turkey.
6. Transfer to a serving plate and serve with some fresh cucumber or tomatoes.

Freestyle Points Per Serving: 11

(Calories 435 | Total Fats 4.1g | Net Carbs: 78g | Protein 16.4g |Fiber: 3g)

Eggplant Rigatoni

 Prep Time: 10 MIN |  Cook Time: 13 MIN | 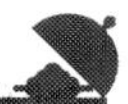 Serves: 6

Ingredients:

For cooking:

1 tsp olive oil

½ cup vegetable stock

For rigatoni:

12 oz rigatoni pasta

1 medium-sized eggplant, cut into small cubes

1 tbsp fresh parsley, finely chopped

1 medium-sized onion, chopped

1 tbsp Parmesan cheese, grated

1 tbsp dry sherry

1 tsp balsamic vinegar

Seasoning:

1 tsp sea salt

½ tsp dried oregano, ground

½ tsp marjoram, ground

1 tsp fresh basil, finely chopped

½ tsp black pepper, ground

Directions:

1. Plug in the Instant Pot and place the pasta in the stainless steel insert. Add water enough to cover all and sprinkle with some salt. Lock the lid and adjust the steam release handle. Press the Manual button and set the timer for 5 minutes. Cook on High pressure.
2. When done, perform a quick pressure release and open the pot. Drain well the pasta and remove the liquid. Pat dry the stainless steel insert.
3. Now, press the Sauté button and add onions. Cook until the onions translucent and then add eggplant. Drizzle with dry sherry, balsamic vinegar, oregano, marjoram, parsley, salt, and pepper. Stir well and cook for 2 minutes.
4. Pour in the vegetable stock and bring it to a boil. Cook for 5 minutes, stirring occasionally.
5. Turn off the pot and stir in the pasta. Transfer all to a serving plate and sprinkle with fresh basil and Parmesan cheese before serving. Enjoy!

Freestyle Points Per Serving: 5

(Calories 207 | Total Fats 2.7g | Net Carbs: 34.4g | Protein 8.2g |Fiber: 3.1g)

Spaghetti Marinara

 Prep Time: 10 MIN |  Cook Time: 13 MIN |  Serves: 7

Ingredients:

For cooking:

1 tsp olive oil
Water

For spaghetti:

1 lb spaghetti pasta
½ tsp sea salt
Water

For Marinara Sauce:

2 cups tomatoes, diced
1 tbsp heavy cream
1 tbsp tomato paste
½ tsp dried thyme, ground
½ tsp dried oregano, ground
¼ tsp garlic powder
¼ tsp dried rosemary, ground
¼ tsp sea salt
½ tsp red chili pepper

Directions:

1. Heat up the olive oil in your Instant Pot on the Sauté mode. Add tomatoes, heavy cream, and tomato paste. Stir well and bring it to a boil. Stir in the remaining herbs and spices. Cook for 3 more minutes and press the Cancel button. Transfer to a food processor and blend until smooth. Place in a large bowl and cover with a lid. Set aside.
2. Now, add 4 cups of water in the stainless steel insert. Add spaghetti and sprinkle with some salt. Securely lock the lid and adjust the steam release handle. Press the Manual button and set the timer for 6 minutes. Cook on High pressure.
3. When done, perform a quick pressure release and open the pot. Drain well the pasta and remove the liquid.
4. Combine with previously prepared marinara sauce and give it a good stir.
5. Transfer to a serving plate and optionally, garnish with some fresh basil or grated cheese. Enjoy!

Freestyle Points Per Serving: 6

(Calories 212 | Total Fats 3.1g | Net Carbs: 37.4g | Protein 8g |Fiber: 0.8g)

Avocado Ziti with Cheese

 Prep Time: 10 MIN |  Cook Time: 13 MIN |  Serves: 6

Ingredients:

For cooking:

1 tsp olive oil
Water

For avocado ziti:

½ ripe avocado, cut into cubes
10 oz ziti pasta
1 small red onion, chopped
1 cup button mushrooms, sliced
¼ cup sour cream, low-fat
1 tbsp Parmesan cheese, grated

Seasoning:

1 tsp fresh rosemary, finely chopped
½ tsp dried thyme, ground
Salt
Black pepper

Directions:

1. Plug in the Instant Pot and place the pasta in the stainless steel insert. Pour in 3 cups of water and sprinkle with some salt. Close the lid and adjust the steam release handle. Press the Manual button and set the timer for 6 minutes. Cook on High pressure.
2. When you hear the cooker's end signal, perform a quick pressure release and open the pot. Using a large colander, drain the pasta and remove the liquid. Place in a large bowl and set aside.
3. Heat up the olive oil in the inner pot over the Sauté mode. Add mushrooms and cook for 5 minutes, or until soften. Add onions and heavy cream. Stir well and bring it to a boil.
4. Finally, add avocado cubes and sprinkle with thyme, rosemary, salt, and pepper. Cook for 3-4 minutes more, stirring occasionally. Turn off the pot and transfer all to a bowl with pasta. Give it a good stir and transfer to a serving plate. Sprinkle with Parmesan cheese before serving. Enjoy!

Freestyle Points Per Serving: 6

(Calories 212 | Total Fats 7.7g | Net Carbs: 27.8g | Protein 7.2g |Fiber: 1.5g)

Zucchini Farfalline

 Prep Time: 10 MIN |  Cook Time: 18 MIN |  Serves: 7

Ingredients:

For cooking:

1 tsp olive oil
1 cup vegetable broth
Water

For zucchini farfalline:

1 medium-sized zucchini, chopped
1 lb farfalline pasta
1 medium-sized parsnip, chopped
1 cup cherry tomatoes, halved
1 small onion, chopped
2 garlic cloves, finely chopped
1 tbsp fresh parsley, finely chopped
1 tsp soy sauce

Seasoning:

1 tsp Italian seasoning
½ tsp dried oregano, ground
½ tsp sea salt
½ tsp red pepper

Directions:

1. Plug in the Instant Pot and add oil to the stainless steel insert. Heat over the Sauté button and add onions and garlic. Cook for 3-4 minutes, or until translucent.
2. Add zucchini, parsnip, and parsley. Sprinkle with Italian seasoning, oregano, salt, and pepper. Stir well and cook for 2-4 minutes more. Stir in the tomatoes and vegetable broth. Bring it to a boil and cook for 5 minutes, stirring occasionally.
3. Remove all to a large bowl and cover with a lid.
4. Now, pour 3 cups of water in the inner pot. Add pasta and sprinkle with some salt. Securely lock the lid and adjust the steam release handle. Press the Manual button and set the timer for 6 minutes. Cook on High pressure.
5. When you hear the cooker's end signal, perform a quick pressure release and open the pot.
6. Mix pasta with zucchini mixture and transfer to a serving plate. Garnish with some cucumber slices and serve immediately.

Freestyle Points Per Serving: 5

(Calories 223 | Total Fats 2.5g | Net Carbs: 39.8g | Protein 8.7g |Fiber: 1.5g)

Alfredo Penne

 Prep Time: 5 MIN |  Cook Time: 11 MIN | 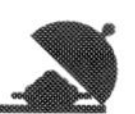 Serves: 6

Ingredients:

For cooking:

1 tsp olive oil

Water

For penne pasta:

12 oz penne pasta

½ tsp salt

¼ tsp black pepper, ground

For Alfredo sauce:

1 cup skim milk

1 small onion, chopped

½ tsp garlic powder

1 tsp all-purpose flour

½ cup cheddar cheese

1 tbsp fresh cilantro, finely chopped

½ tsp dried thyme, ground

½ tsp dried oregano, ground

½ tsp red pepper, ground

Directions:

1. Plug in the Instant Pot and grease the stainless steel insert with olive oil. Press the Sauté button and add onion and garlic powder. Cook for 2 minutes and then stir in the flour. Pour in the milk and bring it to a boil. Add cheddar cheese, cilantro, thyme, oregano, and pepper. Stir well and cook for another 2-3 minutes, or until the sauce thickens.
2. Transfer the sauce to a medium-sized bowl and cover with a lid. Set aside.
3. Now, pour 3 cups of water in the inner pot. Add pasta and sprinkle with some salt and pepper. Securely lock the lid and adjust the steam release handle. Press the Manual button and set the timer for 6 minutes on High pressure.
4. When done, perform a quick pressure release and open the pot. Drain the pasta and transfer to a serving bowl. Drizzle with Alfredo sauce and give it a good stir.
5. Garnish with some freshly grated lemon zest and Parmesan cheese before serving. Enjoy!

Freestyle Points Per Serving: 7

(Calories 234 | Total Fats 5.2g | Net Carbs: 35.2g | Protein 10.4g |Fiber: 0.5g)

Cajun Chicken Risotto

 Prep Time: 15 MIN |  Cook Time: 20 MIN | 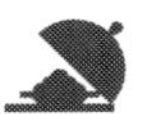 Serves:

Ingredients:

For cooking:

1 tsp olive oil
Water

For risotto:

½ cup rice
7 oz chicken breasts, skinless, boneless, and chopped into bite-sized pieces
2 slices of bacon, chopped
1 medium-sized tomato, chopped
1 red bell pepper, sliced
¼ cup green peas
1 tbsp celery stalks, finely chopped

Seasoning:

2 tsp Cajun seasoning
½ tsp white pepper
2 tsp turmeric powder
Salt

Directions:

1. Place the chicken in a deep bowl and sprinkle with Cajun seasoning and white pepper. Let it sit for 20-25 minutes.
2. Plug in the Instant Pot and place the rice in the stainless steel insert. Add ½ cup of water and sprinkle with some salt. Securely lock the lid and adjust the steam release handle. Press the Manual button and set the timer for 4 minutes. Cook on High pressure.
3. When done, perform a quick pressure release and open the pot. Transfer the rice to a bowl and add turmeric powder. Stir until well combined and set aside. Clean the pot.
4. Now, press the Sauté button and add bacon. Cook for 3-4 minutes, or until crisp. Remove the bacon to a small plate and set aside.
5. Grease the inner pot with olive oil and add chicken. Cook for 5 minutes, or until golden brown. Add tomato, celery, bell pepper, and green peas. Bring it to a boil and cook for additional 3-4 minutes. Turn off the pot and transfer all to a large bowl. Add rice and give it a good stir.
6. Optionally, sprinkle with some finely chopped cilantro before serving. Enjoy!

Freestyle Points Per Serving: 5

(Calories 210 | Total Fats 7.3g | Net Carbs: 17.5g | Protein 16.5g |Fiber: 1.3g)

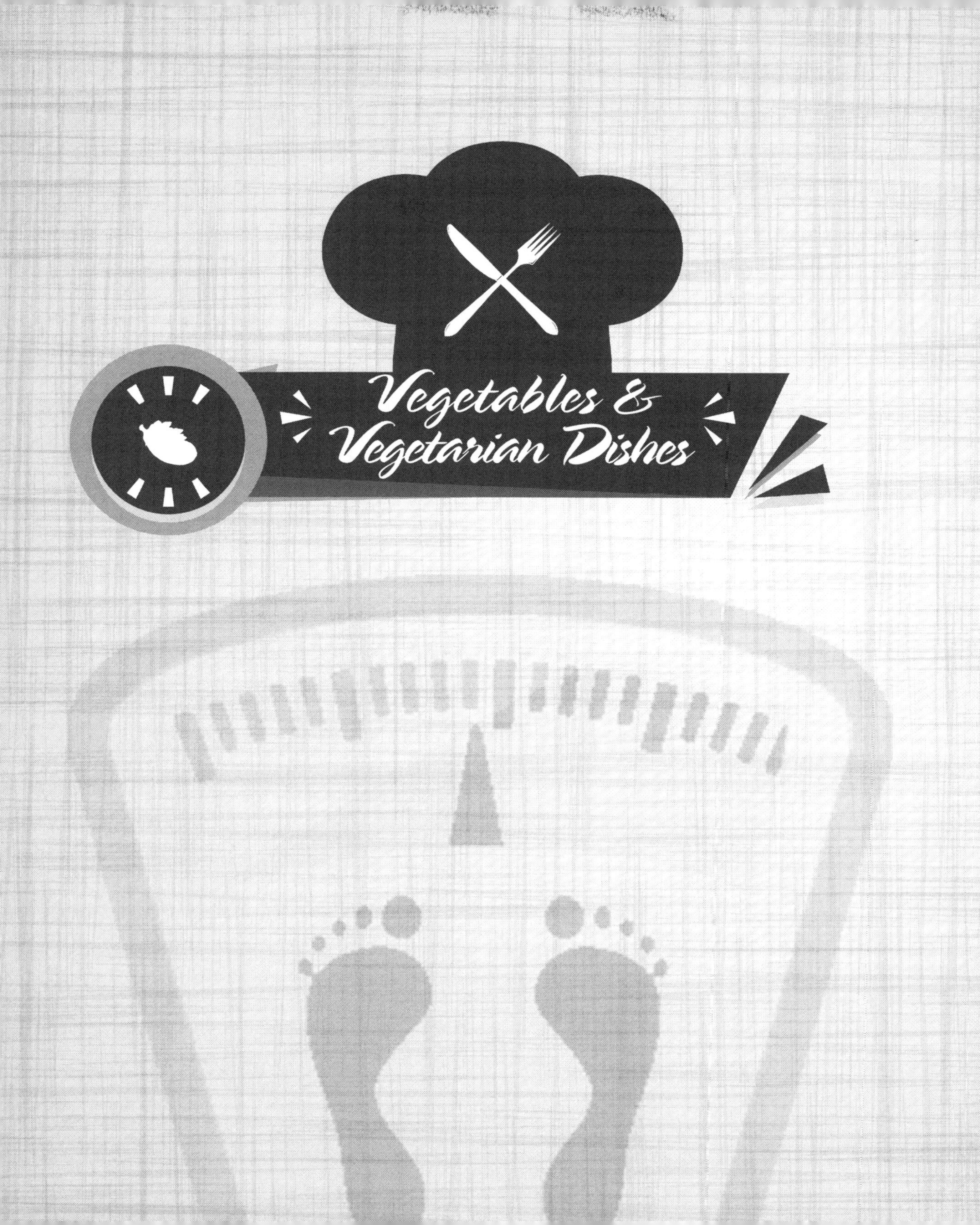
Vegetables &
Vegetarian Dishes

Spicy Asparagus with Cheese

 Prep Time: 10 MIN |  Cook Time: 12 MIN |  Serves: 4

Ingredients:

For cooking:

1 tsp butter
1 cup vegetable broth, low sodium

For asparagus:

1 lb asparagus, trimmed and chopped
1 medium-sized onion, sliced
1 tbsp red wine vinegar
2 garlic cloves, minced
1 tbsp sour cream
½ cup mozzarella cheese
2 tsp fresh parsley, finely chopped

Seasoning:

½ tsp chili powder
½ tsp dried thyme, ground
½ tsp sea salt
½ tsp black pepper, ground

Directions:

1. Plug in your instant pot and place the butter in the stainless steel insert. Press the Sauté button and stir until the butter has completely melted.
2. Add onions and garlic. Cook for 3-4 minutes, or until the onions translucent.
3. Add asparagus and sprinkle with some salt and pepper. Continue to cook for 2 more minutes, stirring occasionally.
4. Now, pour in the vegetable broth and add the remaining seasoning. Stir well and close the lid. Adjust the steam release handle and press the Manual button. Set the timer for 2 minutes and cook on High pressure .
5. When done, perform a quick pressure release and open the pot.
6. Press the Sauté button and stir in the heavy cream and red wine vinegar. Top with cheese and cook for another 2 minutes, or until cheese has melted.
7. Transfer to a serving plate and sprinkle with finely chopped parsley.

Freestyle Points Per Serving: 3

(Calories 71 | Total Fats 2.7g | Net Carbs: 5g | Protein 5.2g |Fiber: 3g)

Broccoli Cauliflower Salad

 Prep Time: 15 MIN |  Cook Time: 11 MIN | 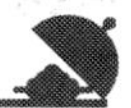 Serves: 3

Ingredients:
For cooking:
Water

For salad:
8 oz broccoli, chopped
8 oz cauliflower, chopped
2 garlic cloves, crushed
½ cup cherry tomatoes, halved
1/2 cup green onions, chopped
1 tsp soy sauce
2 tbsp heavy cream
1 tsp olive oil

Seasoning:
1 tsp fresh mint, finely chopped
1 tsp fresh oregano, finely chopped
Salt
Black pepper

Directions:

1. Place the broccoli and cauliflower in a large colander. Rinse under cold running water and drain. Set aside.
2. Plug in the Instant Pot and pour in 3 cups of water. Sprinkle with some salt and close the lid. Adjust the steam release handle and press the Manual button. Set the timer for 6 minutes and cook on High pressure.
3. When you hear the cooker's end signal, perform a quick release of the pressure and open the pot. Drain the broccoli and cauliflower. Remove the liquid and return the vegetables to the pot.
4. Stir in the heavy cream, soy sauce, garlic, and olive oil. Press the Sauté button and bring it to a boil. Sprinkle with mint, oregano, salt, and pepper. Cook for 2 more minutes and turn off the pot.
5. Transfer all to a large salad bowl and add tomatoes. Give it a good stir and adjust the seasoning, if needed. Let it cool completely before serving. Enjoy!

Freestyle Points Per Serving: 4

(Calories 107 | Total Fats 5.7g | Net Carbs: 7.8g | Protein 4.6g |Fiber: 4.7g)

Quinoa with Eggplant and Lime

 Prep Time: 10 MIN |  Cook Time: 6 MIN |  Serves: 4

Ingredients:

For cooking:

2 tsp olive oil

For salad:

1 cup white quinoa
1 medium-sized eggplant, cut into cubes
1 cup fennel, chopped
1 small carrot, sliced
1 small onion, chopped
1 tbsp fresh parsley, finely chopped
2 tsp fresh lime juice

Seasoning:

1 tsp dried rosemary, ground
½ tsp dried marjoram, ground
Salt
Black pepper

Directions:

1. Plug in the instant pot and place quinoa in the stainless steel insert. Pour in 1 ¼ cup of water and sprinkle with some salt. Securely lock the lid and adjust the steam release handle. Press the Manual button and set the timer for 1 minute. Cook on High pressure.
2. When done, perform a quick pressure release and open the pot. Transfer to a bowl and cover with a lid.
3. Now, grease the stainless steel insert with olive oil. Press the Sauté button and add eggplant, carrot, fennel, and onion. Sprinkle with salt, rosemary, marjoram, and pepper. Stir-fry for 5 minutes, or until softened.
4. Stir in the quinoa, lime juice, and parsley. Turn off the pot and transfer all to a serving bowl.
5. Let it chill for 15 minutes before serving.

Freestyle Points Per Serving: 6

(Calories 238 | Total Fats 5.1g | Net Carbs: 31g | Protein 7.7g |Fiber: 8.4g)

Brussels Sprouts in Lemon Sauce

 Prep Time: 10 MIN |  Cook Time: 10 MIN |  Serves: 2

Ingredients:
For cooking:
1 tsp olive oil

For Brussels sprouts:
12 oz Brussels sprouts, trimmed and halved
1 small onion, chopped
1 garlic clove, minced
¼ cup skim milk
1 tbsp heavy cream
2 tsp all-purpose flour
2 tsp fresh lemon juice
1 tsp lemon zest, freshly grated

Seasoning:
½ tsp smoked paprika
½ tsp cayenne pepper
½ tsp Italian seasoning
Black pepper

Directions:

1. Plug in the instant pot and pour 2 cups of water in the stainless steel insert. Add Brussels sprouts and sprinkle with some salt. Securely lock the lid and adjust the steam release handle. Press the Manual button and set the timer for 3 minutes. Cook on High pressure.
2. When done, perform a quick pressure release and open the pot. Drain the Brussels sprouts and remove the liquid. Clean the pot and pat dry with a kitchen paper.
3. Now, heat up the olive oil in the inner pot over the Sauté button. Add onions and garlic. Cook for 2-3 minutes and then stir in the flour. Cook for 2 more minutes.
4. Pour in the milk and heavy cream. Add lemon juice, smoked paprika, cayenne pepper, Italian seasoning, and black pepper. Stir until well combined and finally, add Brussels sprouts. Cook for 2-3 minutes more and turn off the pot.
5. Transfer to a serving dish and sprinkle with finely chopped parsley and freshly grated lemon zest. Enjoy!

Freestyle Points Per Serving: 3

(Calories 158 | Total Fats 5.8g | Net Carbs: 15.9g | Protein 7.8g |Fiber: 7.3g)

Crustless Vegetable Flan

 Prep Time: 15 MIN |  Cook Time: 6 MIN |  Serves: 4

Ingredients:
For cooking:
2 tsp olive oil

For flan:
1 medium-sized zucchini, chopped
2 small onions, chopped
2 spring onions, chopped
3 red bell peppers, chopped
1 cup cauliflower, chopped
1 cup cottage cheese
¼ cup skim milk
¼ cup fresh parsley, finely chopped
2 large eggs, beaten

Seasoning:
Salt
Black pepper

Directions:

1. In a medium-sized mixing bowl, combine eggs, milk, cheese, and parsley. Mix until well blended. Add all remaining vegetables and sprinkle with some salt and pepper. Stir until all well combined.
2. Plug in the instant pot and grease the stainless steel insert with olive oil. Pour in the previously prepared mixture and securely lock the lid. Adjust the steam release handle by moving the valve to the Sealing position. Press the Manual button and set the timer for 6 minutes. Cook on High pressure.
3. When you hear the cooker's end signal, perform a quick pressure release and open the pot.
4. Transfer to a serving dish and garnish with some fresh cilantro. Enjoy!

Freestyle Points Per Serving: 3
(Calories 173 | Total Fats 6.3g | Net Carbs: 13.4g | Protein 14g |Fiber: 3.4g)

Spring Pepper Salad with Basil Dressing

 Prep Time: 10 MIN | 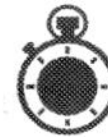 Cook Time: 13 MIN |  Serves: 3

Ingredients:

For cooking:

1 tsp olive oil

For peppers:

1 large red bell pepper, halved lengthwise
1 large yellow bell pepper, halved lengthwise
1 large green bell pepper, halved lengthwise
1 small red onion, chopped
2 garlic cloves, finely chopped
½ tsp Italian seasoning
1 tsp fresh lemon juice
2 tsp fresh parsley, finely chopped
Salt

For dressing:

2 tbsp fresh basil, chopped
1 tsp olive oil
1 tsp red wine vinegar
1 garlic clove, crushed

Directions:

1. In a small bowl, combine all dressing ingredients. Mix until well incorporated and refrigerate for now.
2. Plug in the instant pot and grease the stainless steel insert with olive oil. Press the Sauté button and add onions and garlic. Sprinkle with Italian seasoning, lemon juice, and salt. Stir-fry for 3-4 minutes.
3. Now, add bell peppers and cook for 5 minutes per side, or until charred on the edges.
4. Transfer to a serving plate and drizzle with previously prepared dressing. Let it chill to room temperature before serving.
5. Optionally, garnish with some fresh basil leaves.

Freestyle Points Per Serving: 1

(Calories 81 | Total Fats 3.7g | Net Carbs: 9.9g | Protein 1.7g |Fiber: 2.2g)

Steamed Vegetables

 Prep Time: 10 MIN |  Cook Time: 30 MIN |  Serves: 2

Ingredients:

For cooking:

1 cup vegetable stock, low-sodium

For squash:

2 cups butternut squash, cut into cubes
1 cup cauliflower, chopped
1 cup spinach, chopped

Seasoning:

½ tsp dried thyme, ground
½ tsp red pepper flakes
Salt

Directions:

1. Plug in the instant pot and pour in the vegetable stock in the stainless steel insert. Set the trivet on the bottom of the pot and set aside.
2. Combine squash, cauliflower, and spinach in the steam basket. Sprinkle with thyme, red pepper, and salt. Set the steam basket on top of the trivet and securely lock the lid. Adjust the steam release handle by moving the valve to the Sealing position.
3. Press the Steam button and set the timer for 30 minutes on High pressure.
4. When you hear the cooker's end signal, release the pressure naturally. Open the pot and transfer all to a serving plate.
5. Optionally, drizzle with some lemon juice, balsamic vinegar, or an extra pinch of your favorite herb. Enjoy!

Freestyle Points Per Serving: 0

(Calories 82 | Total Fats 0.3g | Net Carbs: 15.4g | Protein 3g |Fiber: 4.6g)

Creamy Celery Soup

 Prep Time: 5 MIN |  Cook Time: 15 MIN | 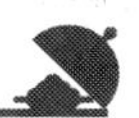 Serves: 5

Ingredients:

For cooking:

2 cups chicken stock, low sodium
1 tsp butter

For soup:

2 cups celery stalks, chopped
1 cup celery leaves, chopped
1 medium-sized potato, cut into chunks
1 medium onion, diced
2 garlic cloves, minced
¼ cup cream cheese, low-fat
¼ cup skim milk
2 tsp all-purpose flour

Seasoning:

¼ tsp cumin powder
½ tsp kosher salt
½ tsp white pepper

Directions:

1. Plug in the Instant Pot and add butter to the stainless steel insert. Press the Sauté button and stir with a wooden spatula until the butter has completely melted.
2. Add onions, garlic, and cumin powder. Stir-fry for 3-4 minutes, or until the onions translucent. Stir in the cream cheese and milk.
3. Finally, add celery and potatoes. Pour in the chicken broth and securely lock the lid. Adjust the steam release handle by moving the valve to the Sealing position.
4. Press the Manual button and set the timer for 5 minutes. Cook on High pressure.
5. When done, perform a quick pressure release and open the pot. Press the Sauté button and stir in the flour. Cook for 2-3 minutes more, or until the sauce thickens.
6. Transfer to serving bowls and garnish with some fresh celery leaves. Enjoy!

Freestyle Points Per Serving: 4

(Calories 109 | Total Fats 5.2g | Net Carbs: 11g | Protein 3.1g |Fiber: 2.1g)

Ratatouille

 Prep Time: 15 MIN |  Cook Time: 18 MIN |  Serves: 3

Ingredients:

For cooking:
2 tsp olive oil

For ratatouille:
2 cups tomatoes, diced
½ eggplant, chopped
1 small onion, chopped
2 bell peppers, chopped
3 garlic cloves, chopped
¼ zucchini, chopped
2 tbsp red wine vinegar

Seasoning:
1 tsp dried marjoram, ground
1 bay leaf
Salt
Pepper

Directions:

1. Preheat the oven to 400 degrees. Line a large baking sheet with some parchment paper and set aside.
2. Dice the tomatoes and spread over the baking sheet in one thin layer. Place in the oven and roast for 10 minutes. When done, remove to a wire rack and set aside.
3. Plug in your Instant Pot and grease the stainless steel insert with olive oil. Add eggplant, onions, bell peppers, and zucchini. Cook for 5 minutes, stirring occasionally.
4. Now, sprinkle with red wine vinegar, marjoram, salt, and pepper. Stir in the roasted tomatoes and pour in ½ cup of water. Securely lock the lid and adjust the steam release handle. Press the Manual button and set the timer for 3 minutes. Cook on High pressure.
5. When you hear the cooker's end signal, perform a quick pressure release and open the pot.
6. Sprinkle with some fresh parsley before serving.

Freestyle Points Per Serving: 1

(Calories 111 | Total Fats 3.8g | Net Carbs: 13.1g | Protein 3.3g |Fiber: 5.9g)

Marinated Broccoli

 Prep Time: 15 MIN |  Cook Time: 18 MIN |  Serves: 2

Ingredients:

For cooking:

3 cups vegetable broth, low-sodium

For broccoli:

1 lb broccoli, cut into bite-sized pieces
1 tsp lemon juice
1 tsp salt
½ tsp black pepper

For marinade:

2 tsp olive oil
1 tbsp dry sherry
½ tsp Worcestershire sauce
½ tsp Dijon mustard
½ tsp dried thyme, ground

Directions:

1. Place the broccoli in a large colander. Rinse well under cold running water. Drain well and transfer to a cutting board. Cut into bite-sized pieces and place in a large bowl. Sprinkle with some salt, pepper, and lemon juice. Set aside.
2. In a small bowl, combine all marinade ingredients. Mix until well combined and drizzle over the broccoli. Toss well and let it stand for 20-30 minutes. Stir occasionally.
3. Plug in the Instant Pot and pour the vegetable broth into the stainless steel insert. Add marinated broccoli with all the remaining liquid. Securely lock the lid and adjust the steam release handle.
4. Press the Manual button and cook for 4 minutes on High pressure.
5. When done, perform a quick pressure release and open the pot. Transfer all to a serving plate and optionally, top with some low-fat cream cheese. Enjoy!

Freestyle Points Per Serving: 3

(Calories 184 | Total Fats 7.6g | Net Carbs: 11.1g | Protein 13.8g |Fiber: 6.2g)

Wild Rice Mushroom Stir-Fry

 Prep Time: 5 MIN |  Cook Time: 12 MIN |  Serves: 3

Ingredients:

For cooking:

2 cups vegetable broth
1 tsp butter

For stir-fry:

8 oz button mushrooms, sliced
1 cup wild rice
½ cup green peas
½ cup celery, chopped
1 small onion, chopped
2 garlic cloves, minced

Seasoning:

½ tsp dried thyme, ground
¼ tsp dried oregano, ground
½ tsp cayenne pepper
Salt
Pepper

Directions:

1. Plug in the instant pot and place the butter in the stainless steel insert. Melt over the Sauté mode, stirring gently.
2. Add onions, garlic, and mushrooms. Cook for 5 minutes, or until the mushrooms soften.
3. Now, add wild rice, celery, and green peas. Sprinkle with thyme, oregano, salt, and pepper. Pour in the broth and give it a good stir. Securely lock the lid and adjust the steam release handle.
4. Press the Manual button and set the timer for 3 minutes. Cook on High pressure.
5. When you hear the cooker's end signal, perform a quick pressure release and open the pot. Press the Sauté button and continue to cook for 3-4 minutes more.
6. Transfer all to a serving plate and garnish with some lemon slices. Enjoy!

Freestyle Points Per Serving: 6

(Calories 278 | Total Fats 3.1g | Net Carbs: 45.8g | Protein 15.3g |Fiber: 6.1g)

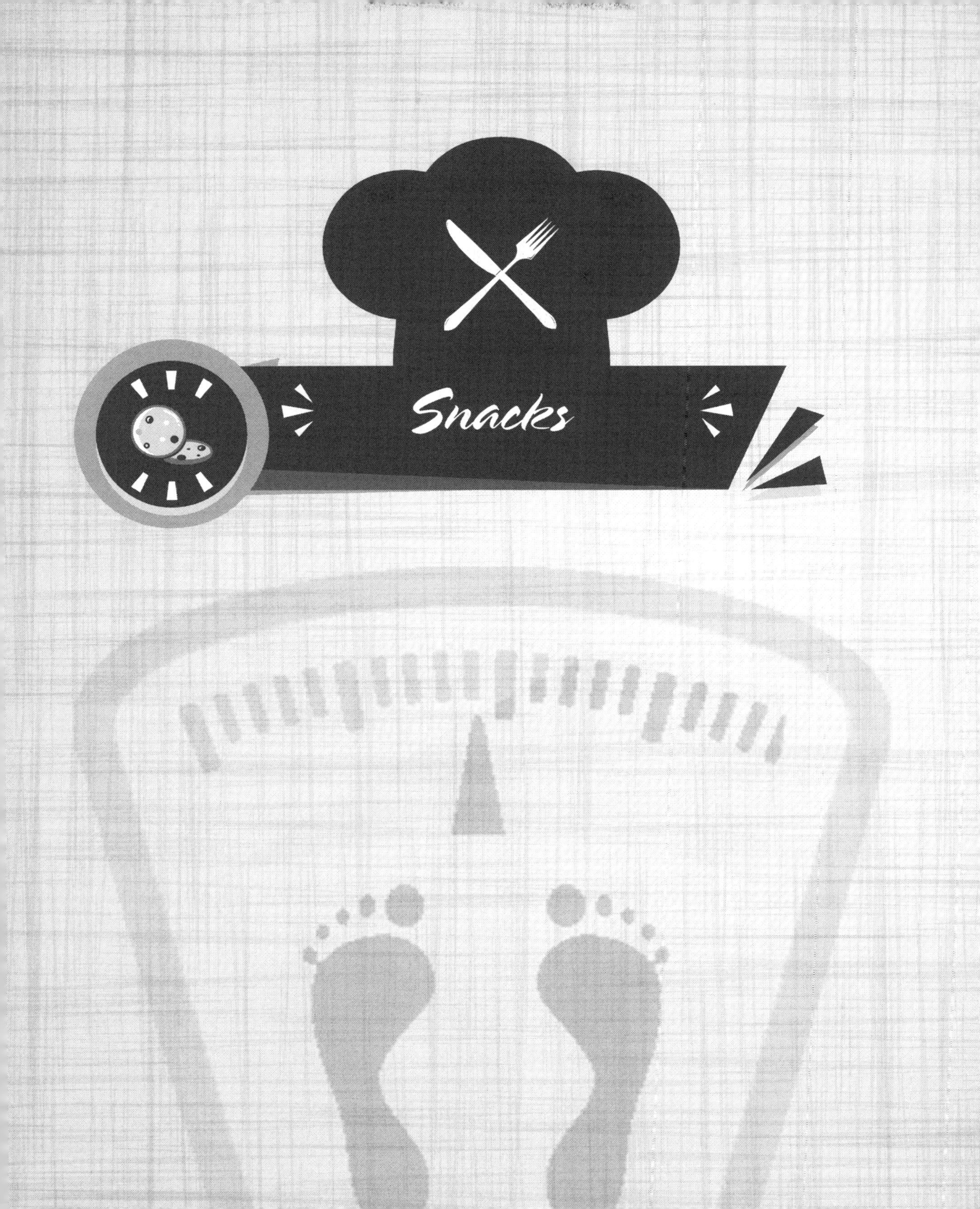
Snacks

Fried Zucchini Toast

 Prep Time: 10 MIN |  Cook Time: 6-8 MIN |  Serves: 2

Ingredients:

For cooking:

1 tbsp olive oil

For toast:

4 slices whole grain bread

½ zucchini, sliced

Seasoning:

¼ tsp dried marjoram

¼ tsp dried rosemary

½ tsp salt

¼ tsp black pepper

Directions:

1. Thinly slice zucchini and sprinkle with salt, rosemary, and marjoram. Set aside.
2. Plug in the Instant Pot and press the Sauté button. Grease the inner pot with olive oil and heat up.
3. Add zucchini slices and cook for 3-4 minutes on each side. Remove from the pot and divide between bread slices.
4. Sprinkle with some more salt and pepper.
5. Serve immediately.

Freestyle Points Per Serving: 6

(Calories 198 | Total Fats 9.1g | Net Carbs: 22g | Protein 6.6g |Fiber: 4.6g)

Vegetable Couscous

 Prep Time: 10 MIN |  Cook Time: 15 MIN |  Serves: 4

Ingredients:

For cooking:

1 tbsp olive oil

For couscous:

1 cup couscous
1 tomato, chopped
1 cucumber, sliced
1 tbsp lemon juice
¼ cup parsley, chopped

Seasoning:

1 tsp salt
½ tsp dried thyme
¼ tsp black pepper

Directions:

1. Place couscous in the pot and pour in 2 cups of water. Add olive oil, salt, thyme, and pepper.
2. Seal the lid and set the steam release handle to the Sealing position. Press the Manual button and cook for 15 minutes on High pressure.
3. When you hear the cooker's end signal, perform a quick pressure release and open the lid. Cool for a while.
4. Transfer to serving bowl and add vegetables. Sprinkle with lemon juice and some more salt.
5. Serve immediately.

Freestyle Points Per Serving: 6

(Calories 209 | Total Fats 4g | Net Carbs: 34.2g | Protein 6.3g |Fiber: 2.9g)

Mini Mushroom Tart

 Prep Time: 15 MIN |  Cook Time: 25 MIN |  Serves: 4

Ingredients:

For cooking:

1 tbsp olive oil

For tart:

10oz spinach, chopped
1 onion, chopped
1 lb button mushrooms, sliced
2 oz cottage cheese
4 (6-inch) pie crust

Seasoning:

Salt and pepper to taste

Directions:

1. Plug in the Instant Pot and press the Sauté button. Grease the inner pot with oil and heat up.
2. Add onions and sprinkle with some salt. Cook for 2-3 minutes.
3. Now add mushrooms and continue to cook until all the liquid has evaporated.
4. Finally, add spinach and season with some more salt and pepper. Remove from the pot and transfer to a bowl. Set aside.
5. Pour in 1 cup of water in the inner pot and position a trivet.
6. Place the pie crusts in 4 mini tart pans and add ¼ of the spinach mixture in each. Scatter the cheese on top and loosely cover with aluminum foil.
7. Place tart pans on the trivet and seal the lid. Set the steam release handle to the Sealing position and press the Manual button.
8. Cook for 20 minutes on high pressure.
9. When done, release the pressure by moving the pressure valve to the Venting position.
10. Open the lid and carefully remove the tart pans. Cool to room temperature and serve.

Freestyle Points Per Serving: 6

(Calories 168 | Total Fats 8.1g | Net Carbs: 15.7g | Protein 8.5g |Fiber: 3.5g)

Warm Gazpacho

 Prep Time: 10 MIN |  Cook Time: 3-4 MIN |  Serves: 2

Ingredients:

For cooking:

1 tbsp olive oil
½ tsp sherry vinegar
¼ tsp red wine vinegar

For tart:

2 tomatoes, chopped
2 bell peppers, chopped
2 cucumbers, sliced
1 garlic clove, minced
¼ cup cottage cheese

Seasoning:

Salt and pepper to taste

Directions:

1. Place tomatoes in a food processor and puree until smooth.
2. Add the remaining ingredients and process until mostly smooth. Set aside.
3. Plug in the Instant Pot and press the Sauté button. Pour in the tomato mixture and season with salt and pepper.
4. Cook for 3-4 minutes.
5. Press the Cancel button and stir in the cheese.
6. Mix well and serve immediately.

Freestyle Points Per Serving: 5

(Calories 193 | Total Fats 8.4g | Net Carbs: 21.7g | Protein 8.2g |Fiber: 4.6g)

Easy Spinach and Cheese Pizza

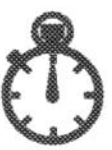 Prep Time: 20 MIN | 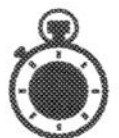 Cook Time: 25 MIN | 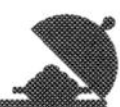 Serves: 4

Ingredients:

For cooking:

1 tbsp olive oil

For pizza:

2 cups spinach, torn

1 cup mozzarella, sliced

3 tbsp tomato paste

1 pizza crust

Seasoning:

¼ tsp garlic powder

¼ tsp dried oregano

½ tsp salt

¼ tsp coconut sugar

¼ tsp white pepper

Directions:

1. Plug in the Instant Pot and press the Sauté button. Add tomato paste, one tablespoon of olive oil, garlic powder, salt, pepper, sugar, and oregano. Pour in about ¼ cup of
1. water and bring it to a boil. Cook for 2-3 minutes, stirring constantly. Press the Cancel button and transfer to a bowl. Set aside.
2. Roll out the pizza crust to fit into round baking pan. Pour the tomato mixture on top and set aside.
3. Press the Sauté button again and heat the remaining olive oil. Add spinach and sprinkle with salt and garlic powder.
4. Cook until wilted and press the Cancel button. Remove from the pot and sprinkle over the pizza crust. Top with mozzarella and loosely cover with aluminum foil. Set aside.
5. Position a trivet at the bottom of the inner pot and pour in 1 cup of water. Place the baking pan on top and seal the lid.
6. Set the steam release handle and press the Manual button. Cook for 15 minutes on High pressure.
7. When done, perform a quick pressure release and open the lid. Remove the pizza from the pot and serve immediately.

Freestyle Points Per Serving: 3

(Calories 103 | Total Fats 5.4g | Net Carbs: 9.7g | Protein 4.2g |Fiber: 1.1g)

Spinach Fritters

 Prep Time: 15 MIN |  Cook Time: 10 MIN |  Serves: 6

Ingredients:

For cooking:

1 tbsp olive oil

For fritters:

1 cup pumpkin puree
2 cups spinach, chopped
1 onion, chopped
2 garlic cloves, crushed
¼ cup parmesan cheese
¼ cup cottage cheese
¼ cup all-purpose flour
3 eggs

Seasoning:

½ tsp dried thyme
Salt and pepper to taste

Directions:

1. Plug in the Instant Pot and press the Sauté button. Grease the inner pot with oil and heat up.
2. Combine the ingredients in a bowl and mix well with your hands. If necessary, add some more flour.
3. Shape patties, about 1 ½ inch in diameter. Carefully place in the pot and cook for 5 minutes on one side.
4. Flip over and continue to cook for a couple of minutes more.
5. Serve immediately.

Freestyle Points Per Serving: 3

(Calories 108 | Total Fats 5.2g | Net Carbs: 8.2g | Protein 6g |Fiber: 2g)

Spinach Sandwich with Raisins

 Prep Time: 10 MIN |  Cook Time: 10 MIN |  Serves: 2

Ingredients:

For cooking:

1 tbsp olive oil

For sandwich:

2 slices whole grain bread
1 cup spinach, chopped
3 eggplant slices, about ½ inch thick
2 tbsp Mascarpone cheese
1 tbsp raisins

Seasoning:

¼ tsp salt
½ tsp dried marjoram

Directions:

1. Sprinkle eggplant slices with salt and place in a large sieve. Let it sit for 10 minutes.
2. Meanwhile, plug in the Instant Pot and press the Sauté button. Heat up the oil and add spinach. Cook until wilted.
3. Remove from the pot and set aside.
4. Rinse eggplant slices and gently squeeze with your hands. Add to the pot and cook for 3-4 minutes on each side. Remove from the pot and set aside.
5. Spread one tablespoon of Mascarpone over each bread slice and top with spinach and eggplant.
6. Sprinkle with raisins and serve immediately.

Freestyle Points Per Serving: 6

(Calories 169 | Total Fats 10.1g | Net Carbs: 14.6g | Protein 5.3g |Fiber: 2.5g)

Vegan Bean Burgers

 Prep Time: 15 MIN |  Cook Time: 6-8 MIN |  Serves: 4

Ingredients:

For cooking:

2 tsp olive oil

For burgers:

½ cup canned pinto beans
½ onion, finely chopped
½ chili pepper, finely chopped
1 garlic clove, crushed
2 spring onions, chopped
2 whole-grain burger buns
½ cup arugula

Seasoning:

Salt and pepper to taste

Directions:

1. Rinse the beans and drain in a large sieve. Transfer to the food processor along with onions, chili pepper, garlic, spring onions, salt, and pepper. Process until almost smooth and transfer to a bowl.
2. Shape 4 burgers.
3. Plug in the Instant Pot and grease the inner pot with olive oil. Heat up and fry burgers for 3-4 minutes on each side.
4. Place one burger in each bun, top with arugula, and serve immediately.

Freestyle Points Per Serving: 6

(Calories 162 | Total Fats 2.8g | Net Carbs: 23.3g | Protein 7.5g |Fiber: 4.7g)

Tomatoes Stuffed with Spinach and Cheese

 Prep Time: 15 MIN |  Cook Time: 10-12 MIN |  Serves: 4

Ingredients:

For cooking:
1 tbsp olive oil

For tomatoes:
4 large tomatoes
4 tbsp buckwheat groats
3 tbsp Parmesan, freshly grated
2 garlic cloves, minced
1 cup spinach, chopped
2 tbsp basil leaves, chopped

Seasoning:
Salt and pepper to taste

Directions:

1. Plug in the instant pot and press the Sauté button. Grease the inner pot with oil and add garlic. Cook for 1 minute and then add spinach. Give it a good stir and sprinkle with salt and pepper. Cook until wilted. Remove from the pot and transfer to a bowl. Set aside.
2. Position the trivet at the bottom of the inner pot and set the steam basket on top. Pour in 1 cup of water and set aside.
3. Slice top ½ inch from tomatoes and scoop out the flesh. Stuff each tomato with the spinach mixture and gently place in the steam basket.
4. Seal the lid and set the steam release handle to the Sealing position. Cook for 5 minutes on the Manual mode.
5. When done, perform a quick pressure release and open the lid.
6. Remove tomatoes from the pot and cool to room temperature before serving.

Freestyle Points Per Serving: 4

(Calories 115 | Total Fats 5.6g | Net Carbs: 13.4g | Protein 5.2g |Fiber: 3.2g)

Sweet Potatoes with Cheese

 Prep Time: 15 MIN |  Cook Time: 15 MIN | 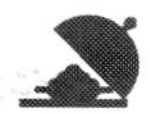 Serves: 6

Ingredients:

For cooking:

1 tbsp olive oil

For potatoes:

2 medium-sized potatoes
1 cup Feta cheese

Seasoning:

1 tsp salt
½ tsp basil, dried

Directions:

1. Plug in the Instant Pot and pour in 1 cup of water. Position a trivet at the bottom of the stainless steel insert and set aside.
2. Line a small round baking pan with parchment paper and set aside.
3. Slice potatoes in half lengthwise to create a pocket. Stuff with cheese and sprinkle with salt and basil.
4. Place in the prepared baking pan and tightly wrap with aluminum foil. Place in the pot and seal the lid.
5. Set the steam release handle and press the Manual button. Cook for 15 minutes on High pressure.
6. When done, perform a quick pressure release and open the lid. Serve warm.

Freestyle Points Per Serving: 5

(Calories 135 | Total Fats 7.7g | Net Carbs: 12.2g | Protein 4.7g |Fiber: 1.7g)

Spring Onion Kofte

 Prep Time: 20 MIN |  Cook Time: 6-8 MIN | 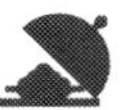 Serves: 6

Ingredients:

For cooking:

1 tbsp olive oil

For kofte:

1 cup mashed potatoes
½ cup white beans, canned
2 spring onions, chopped
4 garlic cloves, crushed
1 tbsp soy sauce
1 chili pepper, finely chopped
2 tsp baking soda
½ cup Feta cheese

Seasoning:

1 tsp salt
¼ tsp basil, dried
½ tsp black pepper
1 tsp smoked paprika

Directions:

1. Grease the bottom of the inner pot with oil and heat up on the Sauté mode.
2. In a large bowl, combine the remaining ingredients and shape 1 ½ inch balls. Gently flatten each with the palms of your hands and cook for 3-4 minutes on each side.
3. When done, press the Cancel button and transfer kofte to a serving plate. Optionally, sprinkle with some freshly chopped parsley or top with Greek yogurt.
4. Serve immediately.

Freestyle Points Per Serving: 4

(Calories 129 | Total Fats 3.3g | Net Carbs: 15.7g | Protein 7g |Fiber: 2.8g)

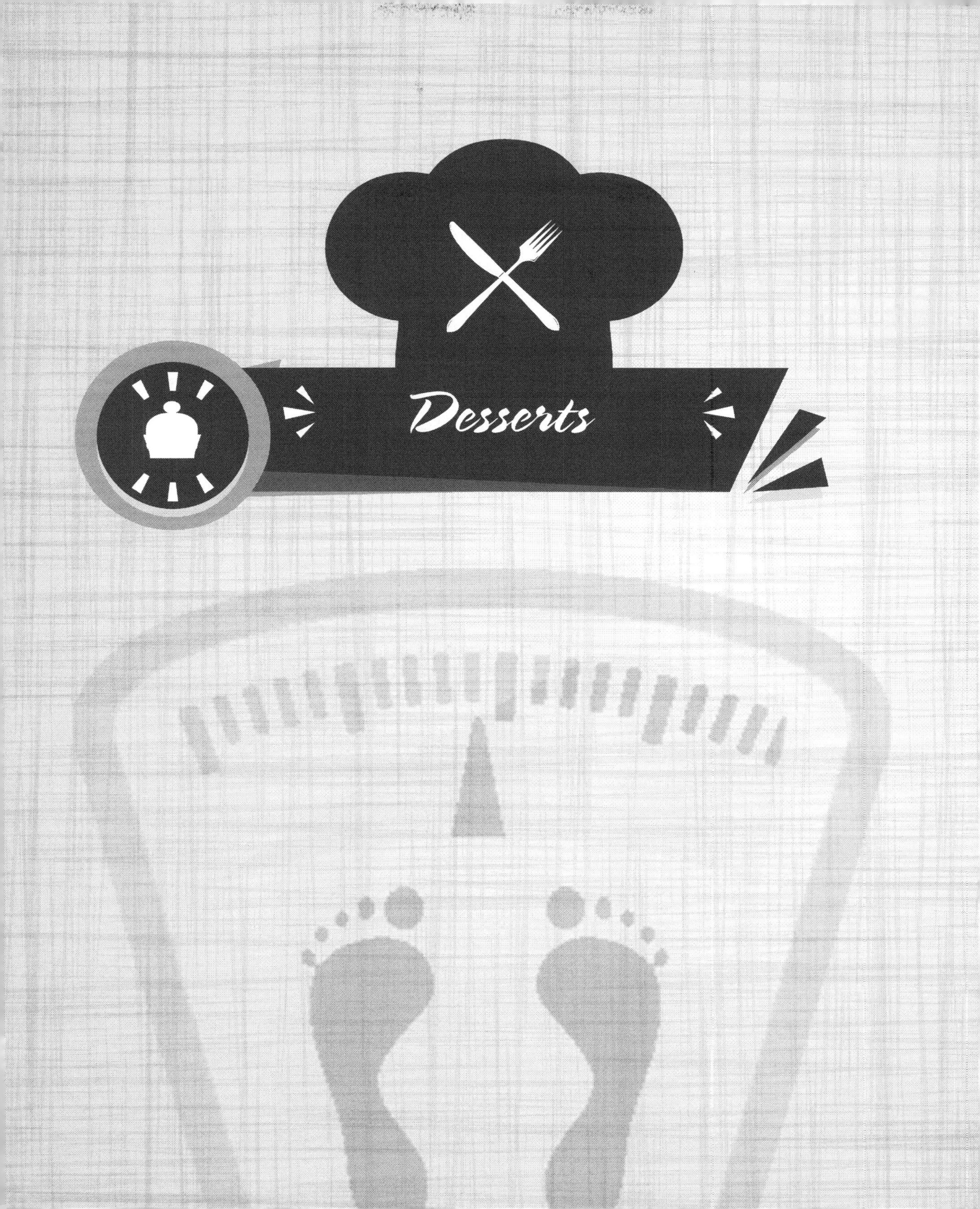
Desserts

Rum Bundt Cake

 Prep Time: 15 MIN |  Cook Time: 40 MIN |  Serves: 10

Ingredients:

For cooking:

Nonstick cooking spray

For cake:

1 cup all-purpose flour
1 tbsp butter, unsalted
¾ cup Swerve
1 large egg
2 large egg whites
5 oz cream cheese, low-fat
½ tsp baking powder
¼ tsp salt
1 tsp rum extract

Directions:

1. Grease a fitting Bundt pan with some nonstick cooking spray and set aside.
2. In a large mixing bowl, combine flour, baking powder, swerve, and salt. Stir until combined and set aside.

1. In a separate large mixing bowl, combine butter, egg, egg whites, cream cheese, and rum extract. Beat with a hand mixer until well incorporated.
2. Now, pour the wet ingredients over dry ingredients and mix until combined.
3. Pour the mixture into the prepared Bundt pan and set aside.
4. Plug in the Instant Pot and pour 1 cup of water in the stainless steel insert. Set the trivet on the bottom of the pot and place the pan on top. Cover the pan with some aluminum foil and close the lid. Adjust the steam release handle and press the Manual button. Set the timer for 40 minutes and cook on High pressure.
5. When done, perform a quick pressure release and open the lid. Transfer the pan to a wire rack and let it chill for a while.
6. Optionally, serve with some Mascarpone cheese and enjoy!

Freestyle Points Per Serving: 4

(Calories 117 | Total Fats 6.7g | Net Carbs: 9.7g | Protein 3.7g |Fiber: 0.4g)

Lime Pudding

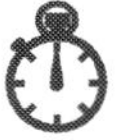 Prep Time: 15 MIN | 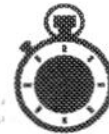 Cook Time: 40 MIN |  Serves: 6

Ingredients:

For cooking:

Nonstick cooking spray

2 cups water

For pudding:

2 oz vanilla pudding mix, sugar-free

1 envelope gelatin, sugar-free

1 tsp lime extract

½ cup Cool Whip, fat-free

Directions:

1. Plug in your Instant Pot and pour in the water.
2. Press the Sauté button and add pudding mix. Bring it to a boil and stir constantly.
3. Now, add gelatin mix and lime extract. Cook for 2 more minutes, stirring constantly.
4. Pour the mixture into serving bowls or ramekins. Let it cool completely.
5. Top each bowl with Cool Whip and refrigerate for 15 minutes before serving.
6. Enjoy!

Freestyle Points Per Serving: 2

(Calories 49 | Total Fats 1.6g | Net Carbs: 7.4g | Protein 1.1g |Fiber: 0g)

Cinnamon Peach Bake

 Prep Time: 15 MIN |  Cook Time: 2 HOURS |  Serves: 4

Ingredients:
For cooking:
Nonstick cooking spray

For peaches:
4 large peaches, sliced
3 tbsp raisins
4 tbsp granulated Stevia
1 tsp cinnamon powder
1 tsp butter

Directions:

1. Wash the peaches and cut into halves. Remove the pits and cut each half into 3 slices. Set aside.
2. Plug in the Instant Pot and grease the stainless steel insert with some nonstick cooking spray.
3. Place the peach slices and raisins in the inner pot. Sprinkle with cinnamon powder and granulated stevia. Spoon the butter on top and securely lock the lid. Adjust the steam release handle by moving the valve to the Sealing position. Set the Slow Cooker mode and cook for 2 hours on Low pressure.
4. When done, release the pressure naturally. Open the lid and transfer all to a serving dish.
5. Chill for a while before serving.

Freestyle Points Per Serving: 2

(Calories 88 | Total Fats 1.4g | Net Carbs: 16.8g | Protein 1.6g |Fiber: 2.6g)

Walnut Raspberry Cookies

 Prep Time: 20 MIN |  Cook Time: 30 MIN |  Serves: 12

Ingredients:

For cooking:

Water

For cookies:

1 ½ cup all-purpose flour
½ tsp baking powder
¼ tsp baking soda
2 tbsp stevia powder
1 egg
1 tbsp cornstarch
¼ cup butter, softened
2 tbsp skim milk
1 tsp raspberry extract
1 tbsp walnuts, chopped

Directions:

1. In a large mixing bowl, combine flour, baking powder, baking soda, stevia powder, and cornstarch. Mix with a spatula until combined and set aside.
2. Add butter and mix with your hands until you get a sandy texture.
3. Pour in the milk and add egg. Continue to mix until well incorporated. Stir in the vanilla extract and mix again until a nice dough has been formed.
4. Line a fitting baking pan with some parchment paper. Spoon about 2-3 teaspoons of dough onto the pan. Gently press with palm of your hand to form a cookie shape. Tuck in the walnuts and set aside.
5. Plug in the Instant Pot and pour 1 cup of water in the stainless steel insert. Set the trivet in the bottom and place the pan on top. Close the lid and adjust the steam release handle. Press the Manual button and set the timer for 30 minutes on High pressure.
6. When done, perform a quick pressure release and open the pot. Transfer the pan to a wire rack and let it cool completely.

Freestyle Points Per Serving: 3

(Calories 104 | Total Fats 4.7g | Net Carbs: 12.4g | Protein 2.4g |Fiber: 0 5g)

Chocolate Mini Fudge Cakes

 Prep Time: 20 MIN |  Cook Time: 30 MIN |  Serves: 8

Ingredients:

For mini fudge cakes:

5 oz unsweetened dark chocolate, roughly chopped
½ cup sugar
6 large marshmallows
2 tsp margarine, reduced-calorie
2 tbsp evaporated milk

Directions:

1. Plug in the Instant Pot and press the Sauté button. Add margarine and milk. Gently stir until the margarine has been completely melted.
2. Stir in the sugar and bring it all to a boil. Cook for 1 minute, stirring constantly.
3. Add chocolate and stir until all well combined and creamy.
4. Turn off the pot and add marshmallows. Stir again until melted. Transfer the mixture into small ramekins and set aside to cool completely.
5. Refrigerate for 1 hour before serving.
6. Enjoy!

Freestyle Points Per Serving: 7

(Calories 138 | Total Fats 6.2g | Net Carbs: 25.5g | Protein 0.7g |Fiber: 1.1g)

Iced Cocoa Brownies

 Prep Time: 20 MIN |  Cook Time: 35 MIN | 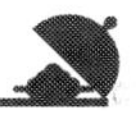 Serves: 10

Ingredients:

For cooking:

Nonstick cooking spray

For brownies:

7 oz condensed milk, low fat
2 tbsp cocoa powder, raw
2 tbsp chocolate chips, sugar-free
2 egg whites
3 tbsp all-purpose flour
½ tsp baking powder
½ tsp cinnamon powder

For icing:

1 cup powdered stevia
1 tbsp coconut cream
½ tbsp skim milk
½ tsp peppermint extract

Directions:

1. Grease a fitting spring-form pan with nonstick cooking spray and set aside.

1. Place the chocolate chips in a small saucepan. Melt over medium-high heat.
2. Stir in the cocoa and milk and cook for 1 minute, stirring constantly. Remove from the heat.
3. In a separate bowl, whisk the egg white, baking powder, cinnamon powder, and flour. Add melted chocolate mixture and combine.
4. Now, pour the mixture into the prepared pan. Shake to flatten the surface and set aside.
5. Plug in the Instant Pot and pour 1 cup of water in the stainless steel insert. Position a trivet on the bottom of the pan and place the pan on top. Close the lid and adjust the steam release handle. Press the Manual button and set the timer for 35 minutes on High pressure.
6. Meanwhile, prepare the icing. In a mixing bowl, combine stevia, milk, coconut cream, and peppermint extract. Mix until creamy.
7. When you hear the cooker's end signal, perform a quick pressure release and open the lid. Transfer to wire rack and let it cool completely.
8. When cooled, spread the icing using a kitchen spatula. Chill in the refrigerator for 1 hour before serving.

Freestyle Points Per Serving: 5

(Calories 93 | Total Fats 2.9g | Net Carbs: 14.2g | Protein 2.9g |Fiber: 0.5g)

Raspberry Muffins

 Prep Time: 5 MIN |  Cook Time: 30 MIN |  Serves: 6

Ingredients:

For cooking:

Nonstick cooking spray

For muffins:

1 cup all-purpose flour
1 tsp baking powder
2 tsp olive oil
¼ tsp salt
1 large egg
5 oz raspberries
2 tbsp milk
½ tsp raspberry extract
1 tbsp dark chocolate chips

Directions:

1. In a large mixing bowl, combine flour, baking powder, and salt. Mix until combined and then add egg, raspberries, oil, milk, and raspberry extract. Stir until well combined and set aside.
2. Grease silicone muffin molds with some cooking spray. Pour the mixture and sprinkle with chocolate chips.
3. Pour 1 cup of water in the stainless steel insert of your Instant Pot. Set the trivet on the bottom and place the molds on top. Close the lid and adjust the steam release handle. Press the Manual button and set the timer for 30 minutes. Cook on High pressure.
4. When done, perform a quick pressure release and open the lid. Transfer the muffins to a wire rack and let it chill for a while. Enjoy!

Freestyle Points Per Serving: 3

(Calories 123 | Total Fats 3.2g | Net Carbs: 18.2g | Protein 3.7g |Fiber: 2.1g)

Orange Squares

 Prep Time: 20 MIN |  Cook Time: 30 MIN | 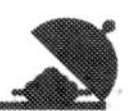 Serves: 6

Ingredients:

For squares:

½ cup all-purpose flour
¼ cup fresh orange juice
2 tbsp powdered stevia
1 tbsp almonds, chopped
1 large egg
1 large egg white
2 tsp vegetable oil
1 tsp fresh orange zest
3 tsp butter
¼ tsp salt

Directions:

1. Combine flour, stevia, almonds, and salt in a large mixing bowl. Mix until combined and then add butter and vegetable oil. Using a hand mixer, beat until sandy texture has been formed.
2. Line a fitting baking pan with some parchment paper. Add the mixture and spread evenly. Press with your hand to form a crust.
3. Plug in your Instant Pot and pour 1 cup of water in the stainless steel insert. Set the trivet on the bottom and place the pan on top. Close the lid and adjust the steam release handle. Press the Manual button and set the timer for 30 minutes on High pressure.
4. Meanwhile, combine sugar, egg, egg white, orange juice, and orange zest. Beat with an electric mixer until smooth and creamy. Set aside.
5. When you hear the cooker's end signal, perform a quick pressure release and open the lid. Transfer the pan to a wire rack and let it cool completely.
6. Pour the creamy mixture over the cake and refrigerate for 30 minutes.
7. Cut into squares and garnish with some extra orange zest.

Freestyle Points Per Serving: 3

(Calories 94 | Total Fats 4.9g | Net Carbs: 8.9g | Protein 3g |Fiber: 0.5g)

Blueberry Mug Cake

 Prep Time: 5 MIN |  Cook Time: 20 MIN |  Serves: 2

Ingredients:

For cooking:

Nonstick cooking spray

For mug cake:

½ cup blueberries
1 large egg
3 tbsp all-purpose flour
2 tbsp cocoa powder, raw
2 tsp powdered stevia
¼ tsp baking powder
¼ tsp blueberry extract
¼ tsp salt

Directions:

1. Combine all-purpose flour, cocoa powder, stevia, and baking powder in a mixing bowl. Mix until combined and then add the remaining ingredients. Beat well until a fine batter has been formed.
2. Grease an oven-safe mug or ramekin with some nonstick cooking spray. Fill about 2/3 of the mug. Optionally, top with some dark chocolate chips.
3. Plug in the Instant Pot and pour 1 cup of water in the stainless steel insert. Set the trivet and place the mug on top. Close the lid and adjust the steam release handle by moving the valve to the Sealing position. Cook on Manual mode for 20 minutes over High pressure.
4. When done, perform a quick pressure release by moving the valve to the Venting position. Open the lid and transfer the mug to a wire rack. Let it cool completely before serving.

Freestyle Points Per Serving: 3

(Calories 112 | Total Fats 3.4g | Net Carbs: 14.8g | Protein 5.6g |Fiber: 2.8g)

Layered Chocolate Mousse

 Prep Time: 20 MIN |  Cook Time: 10 MIN |  Serves: 6

Ingredients:

For cooking:

Nonstick cooking spray

For chocolate layer:

1 ½ cup skim milk

1 tbsp cocoa powder, raw

2 tbsp cornstarch

3 tbsp whipped cream, fat-free

2 tsp stevia powder

For white chocolate layer:

1 ½ cup skim milk

1 tbsp white chocolate

2 tbsp cornstarch

2 tsp stevia powder

Directions:

1. First, prepare the chocolate layer. Plug in the Instant Pot and add milk to the stainless steel insert. Press the Sauté button and heat.
2. Add cocoa powder, cornstarch, and stevia powder. Bring it to a boil and stir constantly. Transfer to a serving cup and let it cool completely. Refrigerate for 20 minutes.
3. Now, prepare the white chocolate layer. Pour the milk into the inner pot and bring it to a boil. Add white chocolate, cornstarch, and stevia powder. Cook for 2 minutes, stirring constantly.
4. Turn off the pot and pour the mixture over cooled chocolate layer.
5. Top with whipped cream and optionally, sprinkle with some cocoa. Garnish with lime or lemon slice.
6. Refrigerate for 20 minutes before serving.

Freestyle Points Per Serving: 3

(Calories 91 | Total Fats 3g | Net Carbs: 10.5g | Protein 4.4g |Fiber: 0.3g)

Strawberry Mini Tarts

 Prep Time: 15 MIN |  Cook Time: 25 MIN |  Serves: 5

Ingredients:

For cooking:

Nonstick cooking spray

For crust:

½ cup all-purpose flour
1 tbsp cocoa powder, raw
1 large egg
2 tsp butter, softened
2 tsp stevia powder
1 tbsp skim milk
¼ tsp salt

For filling:

½ cup strawberries, chopped
1 tsp vanilla extract
3 tbsp cream cheese, low-fat
1 tsp stevia powder

Directions:

1. In a large mixing bowl, combine flour, cocoa, stevia, and salt. Mix well and then add egg, butter, and milk. Beat with an electric mixer until well incorporated.
2. Grease mini tart molds with some nonstick cooking spray. Divide the mixture evenly between molds and gently press with the palm of your hand. Set aside.
3. Plug in the Instant Pot and pour 1 cup of water in the stainless steel insert. Set the trivet on the bottom and place the molds on top. Close the lid and adjust the steam release handle. Press the Manual button and set the timer for 20 minutes on High pressure.
4. Meanwhile, combine all filling ingredients in a medium-sized saucepan over medium-high heat. Bring it to a boil and then reduce the heat to low. Simmer for 3-4 minutes and remove from the heat. Set aside.
5. When done, perform a quick pressure release and open the pot. Transfer the tarts to a wire rack and let it chill for a while.
6. Top with strawberry mixture and enjoy!

Freestyle Points Per Serving: 4

(Calories 102 | Total Fats 4.9g | Net Carbs: 10.6g | Protein 3.4g |Fiber: 1g)

Conclusion

Well chefs, that's it! You hold in your hands everything you need to begin your weight loss journey with the help of your newest pals – the Freestyle™ Freestyle diet and your Instant Pot™! No matter how busy your days may be, these programs work perfectly together to help you incorporate healthy eating into your everyday life for years to come.

They say that it take about a month for a new habit to really stick, but we bet it'll take just one meal for you to fall in love with the endless possibilities of "Instant Freestyle" living! After all, once the stress of cooking and worries over point counting are taken away, what else do you have to lose (besides those added pounds, of course!).

Happy cooking!

Made in the USA
Middletown, DE
25 October 2018